RESTORATIVE YOGA FOR BEGINNERS

MEDITATION AND POSES FOR EASING DEPRESSION, STRESS, ANXIETY, PAIN, AND INSOMNIA

MIA CALDWELL

WWW.MIACALDWELLBOOKS.COM

CONTENTS

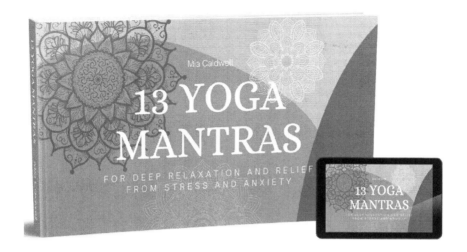

A FREE GIFT TO OUR READERS

Here is a list of my top 13 yoga mantras for relieving stress, free and ready to download right away! This will help you see noticeable results in your mindset, help you actually destress, and change the way you practice yoga forever. Visit this link to receive your gift:

www.miacaldwellbooks.com

INTRODUCTION

When was the last time you were truly still?

Years ago, in my first restorative yoga class, the instructor asked this question. For a moment, I was stumped. I closed my eyes and shifted my weight. When was the last time I had been still? There wasn't an easy answer. Sure, I had spent a moment here or a moment there pausing between hurried activities as I chased my toddler around the house, but actual stillness? Intentional rest? It had been so long I couldn't even think of a time in recent memory that I had given my body a chance to fully relax. As I moved into the pose, the answer hit me with a mixture of shame and disbelief: I genuinely didn't know. It had possibly been years. I would have found the realization funny if it hadn't been so alarming.

Restorative yoga came into my life at a time when I was living in an unsustainable way. As a young mother, I rarely slept, often waking up multiple times a night to check on my daughters. My body was a vehicle I used to get from one commitment to the next. Productivity was my only driving force, propelling me forward from task to task, coffee after coffee, with no thought for my deeper well-being. When I did have time to myself, I would run or lift weights, pushing myself to maintain the incredible warp speed I was living at. In retrospect, I can see now that I was afraid to pause, even for a second. My life was so stressful that I couldn't take a moment for myself to relax, for fear that the world would come crumbling down around me. I was overwhelmed and exhausted mentally, emotionally, physically, and spiritually.

That day, this new, quiet, gentle style of yoga allowed my body to rest and recharge for the first time in years. After that first class, I was hooked. I wasn't sure why, but I knew that I had found a stillness that was missing in my life—a space that would allow me to finally combat the chronic stress I had been holding onto for years. Now, eight years later, I am grateful that this healing, nourishing practice has become a central part of my life. I cannot imagine what my life would look like today without restorative yoga.

Restorative yoga is about carving out a small space in time to take care of yourself. As a mother, wife, daughter, and friend I know how difficult it is to find time for self-care. We are pulled in so many directions with little time to recharge day-to-day. Life is busy, chaotic, and beautiful, but it rarely leaves room for the kind of deep relaxation our bodies need to fully heal. For years, I made excuses to keep myself moving in service of others, but I never extended that same kindness inward. Instead, I kept moving, pushing forward as my body craved rest. My self-esteem suffered and I wrestled with feelings of inadequacy as a mother. I wasn't present for my children because my mind was constantly buzzing, drifting out of the current moment and into the frantic to-do list that the future had become. I was hurting but I was managing just well enough to seem fine on the surface. Inside, I was exhausted, depleted of my ability to truly connect with my loved ones.

Burnout is a serious problem in our culture, even within health-minded circles. We all know how it feels to be exhausted. Between getting the family fed, paying the bills, and vacuuming the house, the need for simple, rejuvenating self-care is higher than ever. Unfortunately, even the act of self-care can begin to feel like a chore if the method you choose doesn't work with your daily schedule. Even something as profoundly healing as meditation or exercise can become yet another bullet point on our daily list of responsibilities if we don't make sure we are giving our bodies the rest they so badly need.

One of the ways that my life was unsustainable before I found restorative yoga was in my constant drive toward perfection. I wanted to be everything for everyone: the best mother, the most thoughtful partner, the caring friend, the savvy professional. This intense need to push myself to the furthest reaches of my potential extended into every part of my life, consuming my self-image. I was so driven to be the best, most flexible, most proficient yogi that I began to lose touch with the deeper, mental benefits of my practice. I lost touch with my ability to be gentle and soft, believing that anything less than perfection was a sign of weakness. Now, I can see how surrendering to the vulnerability of stillness and letting your body pause to rest is a sign of incredible strength.

The yoga community is not immune to our culture's immense pressure to be productive. I am an avid yoga practitioner and I frequently practice more active styles of yoga. While all of these styles hold a special place in my life, restorative yoga provides the backbone of my practice by giving me a break from the hustle of self-improvement. Restorative yoga allows us to be still with ourselves and allow our bodies to be just as they are. This simple, gentle practice can be revolutionary for those of us who don't know how to stop and let ourselves simply be.

Having struggled with my own mental health, I have dedicated the last few years of my life to trying to help others find healing through yoga. As a passionate advocate for mental health, I share my own experiences with restorative yoga so that others who are suffering can begin to heal and become happier, healthier versions of themselves. In my life, this practice has brought me a sense of peace and balance that has allowed me to tackle life's challenges with confidence and compassion. I no longer stumble through life feeling exhausted and critical of myself. This is because restorative yoga has a variety of benefits, both mental and physical.

Because of the unique pacing and postures of restorative yoga, the practice has a profound impact on both mental and physical health. Some of the mental health benefits of the practice include reducing insomnia, improving mood, as well as combatting depression and anxiety. In my own experience, restorative yoga helps me to restore a sense of calm even in the midst of chaos. There are physical benefits, too. It can be used to soothe chronic pain and alleviate digestive distress. Whether an ailment feels rooted in mind or body, restorative yoga allows us to hold space for healing and move forward refreshed. I have experienced this healing capacity myself in profound ways.

Over the past decade, I have spent a great deal of time exploring the history, philosophy, and practice of yoga in all of its forms. I am an avid reader and practitioner, but I started to notice that there aren't enough tools out there to learn the basics of restorative yoga in an accessible, practical way. After years of using restorative yoga to heal my mind and body, I decided I wanted to share what I had learned in hopes of demystifying the practice for others. Often, yoga can feel intimidating for beginners. This book aims to provide simple, easy-to-follow descriptions of restorative yoga postures while providing a strong foundation for understanding how it came to be.

I wrote this book because I am passionate about sharing this practice with others and wanted to provide an accessible guide for beginners. Whether you are a seasoned yogi looking to learn more or a total novice hoping to find a gentle introduction to restorative yoga, I made this book for you. Here you will learn the basics of restorative yoga, including the origins, philosophy, and postures. Throughout the second half of the book, you will learn a series of beginner poses that yield specific benefits—from poses for relieving back pain and poses for eliminating insomnia, to poses targeting anxiety and depression. In addition, I have included sequences to guide your at-home practice and get you started on developing a routine that works for your specific schedule and needs. This book will introduce restorative yoga into your daily life in a way that is accessible, gentle, and simple.

We all deserve to feel at peace, to feel capable of being our best selves. To do this, we need to embrace stillness and allow our bodies to recharge. Welcome to the beautiful practice of restorative yoga. Let's begin.

1

INTRODUCTION TO RESTORATIVE YOGA

WHAT IS RESTORATIVE YOGA?

R estorative yoga is a physical practice focused on relaxing the body, and in turn, the mind. During a restorative yoga sequence or class, students move through a series of long-lasting, still poses designed to let the body's muscles fully release. By relaxing the physical body, restorative yoga allows us to connect with ourselves in a non-judgmental, healing capacity. The use of props is also an essential part of restorative yoga, but these can easily be substituted with everyday household items. By using physical objects to support the body, we are able to experience gentle stretching alongside deep relaxation.

Practitioners of restorative yoga come from all walks of life and all ages and ability levels. Because the practice is so gentle and slow-moving, it is an ideal entry point to yoga for people who are limited in their mobility. Restorative yoga is a wonderful practice for people with chronic illness or pain, as well as those struggling with mental wellness issues such as insomnia, stress, or depression. If you are new to yoga, restorative yoga is a simple entry point into the practice that gives you a solid foundation in terms of yoga's physical, emotional, and spiritual benefits. Due to the gentle, accessible nature of restorative yoga, it is a rare physical activity that can be sustained throughout a person's entire lifespan; whether you are an anxious teenager, an arthritic elder, or a pregnant woman experiencing the discomforts of carrying a child, developing a restorative yoga practice is possible and sustainable.

In my own life, restorative yoga had a revolutionary impact on my ability to let myself rest. So often, we push ourselves to do a million things at once. Our lives are so busy that true stillness and rest are hard to come by. Our culture is set up in a way that disconnects us from our own bodies and forces us to disregard our emotional, mental, and spiritual well-being. In my own life, restorative yoga has let me connect with myself and attend to my body's needs in a way I had never been taught to do previously.

The first time I took a restorative yoga class, I fell asleep. At the end of the class, I woke up, nervous that I would be in trouble and terrified that I had been disruptive in my accidental napping. Instead, the instructor was supportive and encouraging. The way she reacted made me pause and think. She showed me that it is okay to let yourself rest when you need to recuperate—an idea that was simple and yet I had never considered it before.

We live in a world that prizes productivity and progress. Multitasking is seen as a virtue, with every other blogger sharing their advice for how to be more efficient, or how to juggle countless side hustles on top of your daily work. This culture of speed and progress often leaves us exhausted in ways that are deep-reaching and profound. Working hard is always celebrated, but what many of us need is permission to do the exact opposite.

THE HISTORY AND PHILOSOPHY OF RESTORATIVE YOGA

Restorative yoga emerged in the San Francisco Bay Area in the early 2000s through the work of yoga teacher Judith Hanson. Hanson was a former student of famed yogi B.K.S. Iyengar, a prolific yoga educator who is widely considered one of the fathers of modern yoga.

The philosophy of Iyengar was to make yoga accessible to everyone through a focus on eliminating pain and discomfort during practice. Iyengar's form of yoga spread across North America, becoming one of the most widely practiced styles still being taught today. In Iyengar yoga, props are widely used and practitioners are encouraged to pay close attention to their bodies as they move through each pose. Hanson took Iyengar's philosophy further by creating a yoga practice aimed at relaxation and healing, that was accessible to all people, not only those who are already healthy or able-bodied. Restorative yoga emerged as a practice that is possible for everyone, from seriously ill cancer patients to marathon runners looking for a relaxation practice to complement their vigorous fitness routines.

HOW DOES RESTORATIVE YOGA WORK?

Restorative yoga works. There is no debate that the practice is an effective way to promote health and well-being. The interesting question to explore is *why*. There is a lot of evidence to support the practice from both traditional holistic and western scientific perspectives. Often, people fall into the trap of either viewing yoga from an esoteric, spiritual outlook, or a scientific, fitness outlook. This does not have to be the case, as these ways of seeing the practice add depth and layers to its history and effectiveness.

In my own life, I have found it beneficial to view these understandings as complementary ways of explaining why yoga works. They do not need to contradict, as both ways of understanding yoga's benefits add deeper layers of meaning to the practice. Restorative yoga, in particular, is healing in ways that scientific evidence has confirmed and that continue to resonate with traditional yoga philosophies. In the following sections, I will explain multiple ways of understanding restorative yoga and why it works so well as a healing modality.

Scientific Perspective: Understanding the Nervous System

Understanding the nervous system is central to understanding why and how restorative yoga is such a powerfully relaxing and healing practice. Our bodies are filled with neural pathways that help us to perform daily tasks, such as breathing or walking. These pathways are an intricate, endless superhighway of information, travelling at warp speed between our brain and our body throughout our lives.

One large part of our nervous system is the autonomic nervous system, the part of our elaborate neural anatomy that controls our unconscious functions, allowing us to do things like inhale and exhale without conscious effort. The autonomic system is also responsible for our blood pressure and heart rate, central pieces of our daily physical experiences that often feel beyond our control and dictate our comfort levels moment to moment. A racing heart rate can make you feel tense, agitated, and anxious. Low blood pressure, on the other hand, can make us feel drowsy, detached, and unmotivated. Our nervous system is deeply linked to our emotional experience of the world around us.

In order to understand how restorative yoga works on our nervous system to produce healing and relaxation effects, it is important to understand how our nervous system operates. Our autonomic nervous system is split into two main parts: the sympathetic nervous system and the parasympathetic nervous system. The sympathetic nervous system is responsible for reacting to stress as we move through the world. When we encounter a rude coworker or misplace our keys, our sympathetic nervous system increases our heart rate and blood pressure, giving us the boost in energy needed to tackle challenges and meet threats head-on. Without this system, we would be lost in the face of danger. Our sympathetic nervous system keeps us alert and triggers our fight or flight response when we sense that something is amiss. In this way, we need our sympathetic nervous system to keep us safe from real harm.

The other half of our autonomic nervous system is the parasympathetic nervous system. This system is responsible for turning off the fight or flight response and returning our bodies to a resting state, where we are able to relax, digest, and recover from the strains of the day. This system is turned on when we feel safe and free from danger. In an ideal world, the two parts of our autonomic nervous system should work together in harmony, taking turns activating and switching off as we encounter and recover from stressful events. Unfortunately, this isn't always the case for most people.

Life in the twenty-first century is inherently stressful. Between the demands of our jobs and the overwhelming information we encounter daily, we spend our lives immersed in stressors that our body interprets as threats to our safety. Therefore, our sympathetic nervous systems are often left turned on long after any real danger, perceived or legitimate, has passed. The chronic stress of bills, traffic, and chores often cause our systems to operate on overdrive, raising our baseline adrenaline to levels better suited for truly life or death situations. Because of this, many of us walk around all day on edge, unable to ever truly unwind because our bodies are convinced we are in real, physical danger. Without intervention, heightened stress levels can lead to serious disease long-term. In addition, our parasympathetic nervous systems cannot do their job if we are constantly living in a state of perpetual stress and worry.

This is where restorative yoga can help. The goal of restorative practice is to activate our parasympathetic nervous systems through stillness and deep breathing. By gently embracing simple, calming postures, we can help our bodies transition out of stress responses and into relaxation and healing. This is why restorative yoga has such a powerful impact on our bodies. It may initially seem counterintuitive that restorative yoga has been found to lead to weight loss or improved digestion for some practitioners, but the connection is clear once you have an understanding of the nervous system. Using props, stillness, and breath to guide ourselves into a calmer state helps us to trigger our parasympathetic nervous system and move out of fight or flight. In doing so, we improve our ability to recuperate and digest. Once we are in a parasympathetic state, we are more able to heal ourselves and process our emotions.

Restorative yoga has a very real, tangible impact on our health as it encourages our bodies to heal themselves from the problems caused by chronic daily stress as well as deeper, more acute trauma. We often forget that our bodies are capable of healing themselves if we allow them the time and space to do so. Restorative yoga does just this.

Spiritual Perspectives

Modern restorative yoga has emerged from a variety of ancient Hindu traditions, as well as philosophical under-standings that predate the religion and cultural framework of Hinduism altogether. In this section, I will give you a brief overview of the belief systems that make restorative yoga what it is today.

It's important to remember that, regardless of your own beliefs, yoga comes from a rich historical background. Understanding the meaning behind yoga will help you deepen your practice as you dive into the amazing world of restorative yoga. These concepts are enormous and complex, so I have summarized them here in simple terms.

Ayurveda

Ayurveda is the medical system that operates alongside yoga in traditional Indian culture. Ayurvedic wisdom places each of us into three constitutions, or doshas, which describe our essential nature. Each dosha comes with specific recommendations for physical yogic practice, as well as dietary needs and other important parts of daily life. The three doshas are kapha, pitta, and vata.

Those who fit into the vata dosha category tend to be caught up in their thoughts. They are prone to anxiety and over-thinking, along with frequent digestive issues due to their worrying nature. If you find yourself unable to turn off your thoughts and experience difficulty sitting still, you may be vata. Restorative yoga is a profoundly helpful practice for people who fall into this category, as it allows them to let go of their daily worries and simply be in the present moment.

Pitta dosha, on the other hand, is the category for ambitious, driven, fiery people. Like vata dosha, pitta people are always in motion, whether physically or mentally. They work incredibly hard and have a hard time slowing down to relax, as they have big goals and see leisure time as wasted opportunities. In today's busy, productivity-focused world, pitta people rarely take time to let go of their lofty goals to simply sit back and relax. Restorative yoga is essential to help pitta people add healthful balance to their regimented, purpose-driven lives.

Finally, kapha dosha is the third, less adrenaline-driven dosha. People who fit into this final category actually benefit from adding more motion to their daily lives, as kapha comes with a tendency for stillness, indecision, and apprehension. There is a common misconception that slower forms of yoga are not as beneficial for kapha people, but this is actually far from the truth. Everyone requires a balance of motion and stillness in their lives, making restorative yoga a valuable practice for us all, regardless of our natural inclinations.

The Five Koshas

In traditional yogic philosophy, our existences can be thought of as five interconnected layers, each one deeper and more profound than the last. These layers are called the koshas. Knowing each of these layers allows us to be more connected to our innermost self. Yoga allows us to experience each of these layers and achieve a sense of peaceful balance.

Our experiences begin in the physical realm, which is referred to as **the annamaya-kosha**. This layer of existence is where we experience physical sensations and it is associated with the earth element. Our annamaya-kosha is the surface of our existence and the site of our physical health, including diet and exercise. By keeping this layer healthy, we allow ourselves to connect with the deeper, less visible koshas.

Next is **the pranamaya-kosha.** This layer is our vital life energy, which flows throughout the body, weaving throughout the annamaya-kosha. Associated with the water element, our pranamaya-kosha is commonly thought of as an aura, but it also includes energetic pathways and meridians throughout the physical body. When we take in breath, food, and other forms of energy, we replenish our life energy. An awareness of this system helps us to connect with ourselves on a deeper level beyond merely the physical.

After the annamaya- and pranamaya-koshas is the third layer, associated with the fire element: **the manomaya-kosha**. This layer is home to our emotions and our thoughts, which interact with the previous two layers to add meaning to our experiences. When we become more mindful and aware of our judgments and feelings, we can connect with this layer of existence and enhance our ability to feel peaceful and balanced. The goal of yoga is to increase our awareness of the ways that these layers of existence interact and to make space for ourselves to exist peacefully alongside our feelings rather than try to fight against them.

Woven throughout these first three layers, **our vijnana-maya-kosha** is our innate wisdom and intuition. This layer is associated with the air element, as it is a subtle, yet powerful layer of our experiences. Known in many cultures as our inner voice, this layer is the site of our intuitive connection with the universe. When we connect with the first three koshas and find harmony, we are able to hear our vijnanamaya-kosha and access wisdom that comes from forces beyond ourselves. This layer is where we can begin to see the interconnectedness of all things and appreciate the deeper lessons that life has to offer.

Finally, the last, deepest layer of our koshas is the state of bliss, **the anandamaya-kosha,** associated with space, or the ether. As we peel back each layer of our own experiences, we get closer to this state of inner peace and permeating joy. In practicing yoga, we can bring ourselves closer to this inner-most, subtle layer of human existence. Restorative yoga, in particular, can give us the space to examine each of these layers and connect with ourselves on a deeper plane.

Chakras

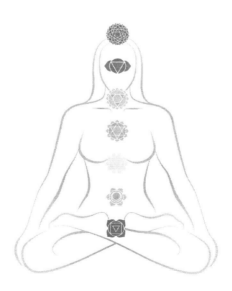

One of the most incredible ways that eastern and western understandings of yoga intersect is through the chakras. In Sanskrit, chakra means wheel or disk, which is a helpful way to view chakras as churning wheels of lifeforce. These energetic points along the midline of the body correspond with specific nerve bundles along the spinal column, linking chakras to scientific understandings of the central nervous system. In traditional yoga, poses allow the practitioner to unblock these energetic wheels and experience a balanced, aligned flow of energy. There are seven main chakras, although many people believe there are upward of one hundred of these points within the body.

Root Chakra – Muladhara

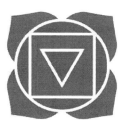

The root chakra, known as the Muladhara, is located at the base of the spine. Our root chakra is responsible for our sense of security and stability in life as we encounter challenges. Having an unblocked root chakra helps us to feel grounded and steadfast when life gets chaotic or overwhelming.

Sacral Chakra – Svadhisthana

Above the root chakra is our sacral chakra, also known as the Svadhisthana. This chakra is where our sensual and erotic energy resides. It is common for people to mistake this chakra for being purely sexual, but it is actually where our creativity dwells. An unblocked sacral chakra allows us to connect to our own emotions and to empathize fully with others. When we are able to let energy flow through this chakra, we are better able to express ourselves through artistic outlets.

Solar Plexus Chakra – Manipura

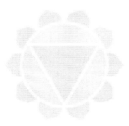

The next chakra along the midline is the solar plexus chakra, known as the Manipura. This chakra is located in the stomach, just below the bottom of the sternum. The Manipura is the home of our confidence and self-esteem, responsible for whether or not we feel like we are at the steering wheel in our own lives. When this chakra is unblocked, we can make decisions with conviction and trust our own choices.

Heart Chakra – Anahata

Above the solar plexus chakra is the heart chakra. In Sanskrit, this chakra is known as Anahata, the site of our compassion, empathy, and love. Freeing up the energy that flows through this chakra helps us to feel connected to others and emotionally aware. When our Anahata is clear, we feel compassion for all living things, including our enemies or people who disagree with us. Clearing this chakra brings harmony into our lives and allows us to feel joyful kindness for others.

Throat Chakra – Vishuddha

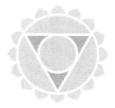

The Vishuddha, or throat chakra, is the wheel of energy that dictates our ability to communicate ourselves in words. When this chakra is blocked, we struggle to make our voices heard and find it hard to articulate our thoughts out loud. Unblocking the throat chakra leads to better verbal communication and helps us find our voice in the face of challenges.

Third Eye Chakra – Ajna

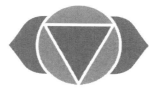

The second to last chakra along the midline is the third eye or the Ajna. This chakra is responsible for our intuition and inner wisdom. A clear third eye chakra lets us see new possibilities and follow our gut instinct in difficult situations. It speaks to us when we need guidance.

Crown Chakra – Sahasrara

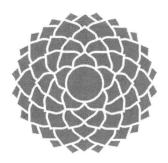

Sahasrara, the crown chakra, is the final chakra along the midline of the body, located on the crown of the head. This chakra is where we connect to our higher purpose in life and access our spirituality. When our Sahasrara is unblocked and energy flows freely, we can connect with forces beyond ourselves and feel at one with the universe.

The goal of yoga is to help our energy to flow freely through each of these energetic points. In my own practice, I have found that paying attention to my chakras during practice helps me to feel more present and mindful in my movements and breath. When we are empowered to understand how these points operate, we can train ourselves to feel more grounded, connected, and calm in our daily lives.

The Eight Limbs of Yoga

As a practice, yoga has been around for thousands of years. An ancient text called the Yoga Sutras by a writer named Patanjali outlines eight parts of the practice. By focusing on each of these "limbs" practitioners can experience all the benefits that yoga has to offer. These limbs work their way from the outer world to the inner world of the individual as they grow closer to a fully realized, enlightened state.

1. Yama

Yama is a word that roughly means control or restraint in Sanskrit. In the context of the eight limbs of yoga, yama refers to gaining control over your impulses and desires so that you can interact with the world correctly. This limb of yoga contains the five principles for living ethically in the world: nonviolence, truth, non-stealing, right use of energy, and non-attachment. By following these principles, practitioners remain on the path toward enlightenment.

2. Niyama

Like the yamas, there are five niyamas. These principles offer a guide for how to interact properly with your own inner self: physical purity, contentment, devotion, endurance, and self-awareness. By practicing each of these principles, yogis bring themselves closer to a peaceful, balanced state of being.

3. Asana

In North America and Europe, when we talk about yoga, we are most often referring to asana, or physical, pose-based yoga. Here, asana simply means the way we sit when we practice meditation. The focus of this limb is to find a seated posture that feels comfortable enough for you to practice total stillness for an extended period of time. Over the centuries, practitioners have expanded this limb to include physical yoga in all of its various forms.

4. Pranayama

Pranayama is the Sanskrit word that means both breath control and breath freedom. This dual meaning is how we understand breathwork as the practice of both controlling our breath and letting it go completely. In yoga, breath is understood as a vital life force. Therefore, having more of a connection with our breath is another stepping stone on the path to enlightenment.

5. Pratyahara

This limb refers to the ability to turn inward during meditation, focusing only on the subject of your meditation, rather than the sensations around you. This is a challenging skill that many new practitioners work hard at when they first start meditating. When we are able to become fully engrossed in the present moment, we are able to bring this skill into our everyday lives.

6. Dharana

Dharana is the sixth limb of yoga. This limb is the power of concentration, or the ability to focus on one thing for an extended period of time.

7. Dhyana

Dhyana is closely linked to dharana and refers to the type of meditation that requires deep mental focus to sustain. Dhyana is only possible once you have fully committed to the previous six limbs.

8. Samadhi

The final limb of yoga is samadhi, the state of enlightenment. When we experience samadhi, we feel an overwhelming sense of peace and joy.

Types of Yoga

Yoga is a practice with many styles and traditions. At its core, yoga is a union between our minds, bodies, and spirits. The goal in yoga is to feel like you are connected, peaceful, and at one with all parts of who you are. In North America and Europe, the most common type of yoga you will encounter is asana, or postural, yoga. Think yoga mats, low lighting, downward dog. Asana yoga is rooted in physical poses and movements, with a philosophical framework that stems from ancient Vedic beliefs and ideas that still influence Indian culture to this day. Today, there are many types of asana yoga, each with different styles, benefits, and purposes. While these styles overlap a great deal, there are a lot of big differences between them, too. In this section, we will go over a brief summary of some of the most popular, well-established forms of yoga.

Hatha Yoga

Hatha Yoga is asana yoga in its simplest form. This style combines pranayama (breathwork), asana (physical poses), and meditation to create a holistic, challenging practice. Hatha is all about balance. This style is gentle but challenging, perfect for those new to yoga or those looking for an everyday practice that builds strength, focus, and flexibility.

Vinyasa Yoga

Another very popular style is Vinyasa, or Flow Yoga. Vinyasa is a fluid practice, focusing on controlled, mindful movement into and between poses. In a Vinyasa class, poses flow continuously from one to the next, providing you with space to explore movement and enter a moving meditation. Vinyasa is perfect for those who love to get moving and want to get outside their minds in a meditative state. While it can seem like an intimidating style, Vinyasa is actually perfect for beginners because it doesn't require that you sit still for very long.

Ashtanga Yoga

Ashtanga is a dynamic, vigorous form of yoga that uses several series of poses. Like Vinyasa, Ashtanga is all about fluid movement and transitions between poses. However, this style is more challenging, offering opportunities for strength-building alongside the meditative aspect of the practice. People who love Ashtanga enjoy the repetitive style because the set sequences make it easy to lose yourself in the process once you become familiar. In addition, Ashtanga is all about personal growth. Practitioners move at the speed of their own breath, pushing themselves to their limits each time they come to the mat.

Yin Yoga

Yin Yoga is a slower practice that is all about increasing flexibility. The focus of Yin is stretching connective tissues, so poses are held for longer than one minute at a time. In a Yin class, it is not unusual to stay in one pose for upward of four minutes, slowly deepening the stretch over time. Yin is surprisingly challenging, especially for those of us who find it hard to sit still in silence. For this reason, Yin can be really beneficial for people with anxiety or those who tend to focus on strength building in their normal fitness routines. While both Yin and Restorative are slower, calmer styles of yoga, they serve different purposes: Yin aims to stretch the body, whereas Restorative aims for deep relaxation.

Kundalini Yoga

Kundalini yoga is a more spiritual practice that focuses on unlocking your life force energy. During a Kundalini class, practitioners chant and sing alongside breathwork and poses. The benefits of this style include increased feelings of joy and connectedness, as well as the physical benefits of exercise and breathwork. This is the perfect practice for people looking for a deeper, more spiritually grounding type of yoga.

Bikram Yoga

This form of yoga gets its name from its founder, a man named Bikram Choudry, who wanted to bring his own style of yoga to North America. Traditional Bikram classes follow his personally designed series of twenty-six poses and are commonly referred to as hot yoga classes. During a Bikram Yoga class, the temperature is set to ninety degrees, so newcomers can expect to sweat a lot. Bikram is a style that can be incredibly challenging, as it pushes practitioners to their limits both in terms of the heat and the rigorous physical poses. This style is perfect for yogis who like a demanding, yet familiar routine.

Iyengar Yoga

Iyengar Yoga is a form of yoga founded by B.K.S. Iyengar. This style of yoga is all about alignment, with a strong focus on creating balance and strength in the body. Iyengar Yoga is firmly rooted in anatomy and prioritizes the safety of practitioners during classes. Instructors are well-trained and provide students with a variety of props to support them in each carefully guided pose. This style of yoga is great for elders and those with chronic injuries or pain because of the emphasis on proper form.

Power Yoga

If you love feeling powerful and strong, look no further than Power Yoga. This style of yoga is all about strength and endurance. Classes are more spontaneous, with an emphasis on flexibility and movement. As you might guess from its name, Power Yoga is all about challenging the body in new, fun ways as you move through the poses in a constant flow. Some studios run heated Power classes, too, making this style highly varied from place to place. This style is perfect for those who want to do a less spiritual form of yoga while getting a great workout.

Sivananda Yoga

Sivananda Yoga is another form with an individual namesake. Founder Swami Sivananda created this style which follows a routine that includes sun salutations, pranayama, and twelve main poses. Simple and effective, Sivananda Yoga is a great starting point for newcomers or those seeking a gentle, spiritual, easy-to-learn practice.

Prenatal Yoga

As you may have guessed, Prenatal Yoga is a practice that focuses on supporting pregnant practitioners across all stages of pregnancy. Many of the poses are designed to help ease pains associated with pregnancy and labor, with ample attention paid to the hips and low back areas. The focus of this style is on safety and self-care, ensuring that each pose is accessible for women in any trimester. This style is also great for new moms who want to gently begin a physical practice again postpartum.

Acro Yoga

Acro Yoga is a fun, partner-based practice gaining in popularity in recent years. This style relies on teamwork and collaboration throughout each pose, as partners work hard to support one another in the complex, challenging postures. During an Acro Yoga class, one partner acts as the support, or base, while the other partner is lifted into the air as the flyer. This style of yoga is great for couples or those who want to try a more exciting, social practice.

Aerial Yoga

If you are looking for a non-traditional form of yoga and you want to move outside your comfort zone, Aerial Yoga might be for you. This style uses suspended hammocks to support an anti-gravity practice. During a class, practitioners hang upside down in supported inversions. There are a ton of benefits to this type of yoga, including increased flexibility, body-awareness, and circulation.

Physical Benefits of Restorative Yoga

Throughout our lives, we experience many forms of suffering. From illnesses to injuries to the everyday wear and tear that comes with being human, we go through a great deal of stress and pain as we move through the world. Restorative yoga has a wide array of physical benefits that counteract these forms of suffering and help us to remain resilient in the face of new, unexpected challenges.

Often in life, it is hard to hit pause to take a moment for ourselves. Life is fast and demanding, often leaving us in a zombie-like state as we move from task to task. When we allow our bodies to fully relax, they are able to enter into regenerative states. This is why restorative yoga is so powerful: it gives us a specific, dedicated time and space to heal. The importance of rest and relaxation cannot be overstated when it comes to maintaining our physical health.

In this section, we will explore the many physical benefits of restorative yoga. One important thing to remember is that restorative yoga is not a replacement for real medical help for any injuries or illnesses. Instead, it is a helpful, complementary practice that will give your body the proper relaxation it needs to keep itself healthy and strong. By building restorative yoga into your normal routine, you can ensure that you are giving your body a fighting chance to rest effectively.

Restorative yoga calms the nervous system.

As we touched on before, restorative yoga works because of how it impacts our nervous systems. When you practice restorative yoga regularly, you teach your body how to relax by triggering your parasympathetic nervous system and switching off the stress response. Over time, this becomes second nature and your body grows more resilient to the daily stressors you encounter each day.

Restorative yoga enhances flexibility.

During a restorative yoga class, stretching is always gentle and passive, rather than forceful or strenuous. It often comes as a surprise for newcomers to the practice when they discover their flexibility increasing with each session. This is due to the relaxation focus of restorative yoga. Rather than pushing tired muscles to their limits, restorative yoga poses help these muscles to soften, opening up new space in the body slowly over time. After a time, you will likely notice your flexibility increasing as your body becomes accustomed to entering a state of deep tissue relaxation.

Restorative yoga improves digestion.

Experts often refer to the parasympathetic nervous system as the rest and digest system. This is because our bodies ignore our digestive systems when we are under any perceived stress or threat. Have you ever been so worried that you got a stomachache? This is a super common stress response. When we experience a lot of daily stress, be it in the form of parenting responsibilities, social commitments, or even bad traffic, our bodies stop paying attention to our digestion. This leads to all sorts of issues, from constipation to chronic gas, or even more severe chronic issues like irritable bowel syndrome. Practicing restorative yoga allows our bodies to unwind and give our stomachs, intestines, and colons the care and focus they require to properly function.

Restorative yoga relieves pain.

Restorative yoga is a very gentle activity, which makes it perfect for people suffering from issues such as injuries or chronic pain.

By practicing restorative yoga, many people find relief from aches and pains caused by chronic injuries, headaches, arthritis, and back pain. The gentle poses increase your mobility and work to balance tensions that might be causing ongoing discomfort in your body. Many women find that these sessions also help them to deal with cramping caused by menstruation.

Restorative yoga can aid in weight loss.

One of the most counter-intuitive benefits of restorative yoga is weight loss. It seems odd at first, sure. How can an activity be so gentle and still lead people to drop weight? The answer is fascinating. When we are anxious, tired, or stressed, our bodies produce a hormone called cortisol, which causes our bodies to gain weight over time. Yoga, when used for relaxation, has been shown to decrease our cortisol levels, resulting in weight loss. Therefore, lowering your stress through restorative yoga can have an unexpected impact on your waistline and overall health.

Restorative yoga keeps your heart healthy.

In general, yoga is great for keeping your heart healthy long-term. Restorative yoga is great for lowering blood pressure and alleviating stress, both of which contribute to heart problems. Paired with gentle cardio, restorative yoga works wonders to keep your heart ticking away in tip-top condition as you age.

Restorative yoga helps you sleep better.

One of the most profound ways that restorative yoga has helped me is in allowing me the space to fully unwind before bed. I find that I sleep much deeper and longer after practicing restorative yoga, and I'm not alone in noticing this amazing benefit. For people with insomnia, restorative yoga is a great way to train your mind and body to wind down in the hour before bedtime.

Restorative yoga helps you recover from illness.

Another benefit of restorative yoga is that it boosts your immune system. This is because relaxation is important for building effective immunity. When we are stressed, we are more likely to get and remain ill. When we practice restorative yoga, our stress levels decrease and our bodies can get back to repairing and restoring our tissues to a healthy state. Restorative yoga is also a gentle way for those recovering from major illnesses, such as cancer, to begin to safely reintroduce movement and mobility back into their lives.

Restorative yoga gives you energy.

Sometimes when we are exhausted, we shy away from letting ourselves relax for fear that we won't be able to bounce back again. Restorative yoga is a great way to restore your energy by allowing your body to rest enough to feel refreshed.

Instead of grabbing a cappuccino or taking a nap next time you're feeling drowsy or drained, try a quick restorative yoga session. The results will have you feeling rejuvenated in no time at all.

Restorative yoga teaches you to relax.

If you are someone who leads a fast-paced, stress-filled life, it can be hard to flip the switch when you want to take a break. Restorative yoga is a fabulous way to train your sympathetic nervous system to know when it's time to turn on or and when it's time to turn off. If you have anxiety, it can be hard to sit still for long periods, so don't get upset with yourself if it takes you a while to ease into longer and longer poses. Learning to manage stress takes time, which is why building a regular practice is so important.

Restorative yoga supports women during pregnancy.

For many women, pregnancy can be a stressful, unpredictable, and exhausting experience. Our bodies go through so many changes as they prepare to bring a new human into the world that it's no wonder many women end up feeling disconnected from their physical selves as they move through each trimester. This feeling, combined with the risks associated with exercising while pregnant, can lead to a lot of frustration and discomfort. Restorative yoga is a safe, gentle way to stay connected and calm in your body as you move through your pregnancy. In this book, I have included a special section dedicated to pregnancy-safe restorative yoga poses to help women navigate these challenges and experience the benefits this practice has to offer.

Psychological Benefits of Restorative Yoga
Why Mental Health Matters

In more recent years, people have begun to take mental health a bit more seriously here in North America. Still, it wasn't long ago that people were being shamed into silence over mental illnesses like depression, anxiety, or post-traumatic stress disorder. These illnesses are common and impact a growing number of adults in our society, yet we don't often walk the walk when it comes to treating mental health as seriously as physical health.

Ample research has shown that our minds and bodies are more connected than we like to think they are. Studies have shown that anxiety and stress have a profound impact on the gut, contributing to digestive and cardiovascular diseases if left untreated. Consider the last time you felt worried. Where did you feel it? Chances are, you felt the worry creeping in through a subtle tightness in your chest, or a rumbling discomfort churning in your belly. Our bodies hold our feelings and emotions, which manifest themselves frequently through physical symptoms. Like our bodies, our minds can get sick and need help to heal.

How Restorative Yoga Can Help

Thankfully, there is a lot of evidence to show that restorative yoga has a positive impact on our mental health. I have experienced these benefits in my own life, but you don't have to only take my word for it. Countless studies have demonstrated that meditation, yoga, and mindfulness are powerful practices for both assisting in managing mental illness and in maintaining positive mental health long term. As with the physical benefits, it is important to remember that restorative yoga is not a cure-all. Rather, it is a powerful tool for prevention and managing existing issues. Seek proper medical assistance if you are struggling with mental health.

Restorative yoga boosts your mood.

One of the reasons I absolutely crave restorative yoga is the emotional boost it gives me. When I find myself acting grumpy or growing irritable, I know it's time to head to my dedicated restorative space to check in with myself for a while. Restorative yoga feels good and helps us reset our emotional states when we're feeling low. Simply spending a half-hour on my mat recharging helps me to feel less negative day-to-day.

Restorative yoga reduces stress and anxiety.

As we discussed before, restorative yoga calms the nervous system and allows your body to rest. This means that your mind has time to rest, too. Sometimes, when we feel anxious, it's hard to sit still. But, with time, it becomes easier to breathe ourselves into a more peaceful state. This is exactly what restorative yoga, combined with meditation and pranayama, does for me when I'm feeling jittery or worried. Working restorative yoga into your daily routine will leave your mind feeling less frantic and more centered.

Restorative yoga promotes mindfulness.

One of the greatest gifts yoga has to offer has nothing to do with yoga itself. Several months into my yoga journey, I began to notice that the skills I was learning on the mat, such as breathing deeply, noticing sensations in my body, and feeling gratitude for my surroundings, were transferring into my daily life. At the grocery store, I was able to breathe deeply and walk with purpose, unphased by long lines or busy aisles. On walks, I noticed the trees more. I really saw them in their full, incredible detail. Yoga has taught me to be mindful in every part of my life. By practicing restorative yoga, you will teach your body and mind how to be more present in the world. I can tell you from experience that this shift is a profound one when it comes to mental health, as I now approach each day more joyfully, more perceptively, and more mindfully.

Restorative yoga eases symptoms of depression.

One common benefit of regular yoga practice is an increase in feelings of joy and happiness. Many people find that restorative yoga helps them manage their depression symptoms, too! This is in part because depression is an exhausting illness to live with. By giving your body some gentle time to heal, you are giving it the nurturing that it needs to cope with depression. In addition, the focus on mindfulness and gratitude eases other symptoms such as low mood and dissociation, both of which are challenging parts of this mental illness.

Restorative yoga grows your self-awareness.

When you take the time to turn inward and really pay attention to your thoughts and feelings, something really cool happens. You get to know yourself better. Believe it or not, many of us walk around the world not really knowing ourselves on a deeper level. Restorative yoga teaches you to read your body's clues to get a better handle on things like your fears, your desires, and even your triggers. Putting aside one-on-one time for you and your own self is a fantastic way to increase your self-awareness and become a more confident, intuitive person.

Restorative yoga helps you heal from trauma.

For anyone who has gone through traumatic experiences, such as the loss of a loved one, an accident, or a life-threatening illness, it can be incredibly hard to return to life as normal. When we go through traumatic experiences, our bodies don't always know that the threat has passed. For many trauma survivors, it can take a lot of energy to move through the world constantly on edge, fearing for danger to surface. Restorative yoga is helpful for trauma because it teaches your body to return to a state of calm. Often, when we have experienced trauma, our bodies don't feel safe anymore. Restorative yoga helps us to relearn that we are safe from harm, leading to less anxiety and fear as we recover.

From the physical to the mental benefits, restorative yoga has many gifts to offer. In this book, each chapter targets a specific issue to help you use restorative yoga in the face of any challenge. In the next chapter, we will discuss setting up your space for your first restorative yoga session.

2

PREPARING TO BEGIN RESTORATIVE YOGA

Now that you have an introductory understanding of yoga, it is time to prepare yourself to start your restorative yoga practice. Setting up a time and space to build your practice into a long-term routine is actually fairly simple. I have organized this chapter to help you put the pieces together to create your restorative sanctuary in the comfort of your own home. The first step is finding a location where you can fully rest without distractions and interruptions.

Setting Up Your Space

Picture a calming space, somewhere you can fully relax and feel at peace. When I close my eyes, I see a quiet, naturally lit room with wide, open windows overlooking an uninhabited stretch of beach. Do you picture somewhere far from the city, warm and serene? Or, do you picture a cavernous library, with a well-worn, fireside armchair?

When asked to picture the perfect, relaxing location, many of us have a go-to image of a place we have either been to, seen on the screen, or dreamed of visiting. If you're lucky, the place you picture might even be a place within your own home, a private sanctuary of your own making. For the majority of us, though, finding a place to disconnect from the world and let go can be challenging. Fortunately, it is possible to create the perfect relaxation space to practice restorative yoga if you know the right ingredients. In my experience, there are three key ingredients for the perfect restorative yoga space: privacy, lighting, and comfort.

Privacy

One of the most important aspects of a restorative yoga space is that the space feels safe from interruptions. For those of us with busy, hectic lives, it can feel difficult to fully disconnect from the parts of our lives that cause us stress. If you are someone who carries a lot of worry about your daily responsibilities, it can be hard to fully relax if you are reminded of the things causing you stress. This can lead to a pervasive feeling of being constantly on edge, which isn't helpful when you're trying to unwind and let go with restorative yoga.

If you are lucky enough to have a room you can dedicate to your yoga practice, this is not a difficult step to achieve. For the rest of us, I have a few key suggestions for how to build a private space for restorative yoga. First, find a space with a door that closes. Mentally and energetically, closing a physical door to the outside world helps to create a boundary between you and all the parts of your life that might be pulling you away from your practice. It doesn't have to be a room; I have known people who have created small, private spaces in walk-in closets, bedrooms, or even storage spaces. Identifying a dedicated location for your practice will help you to feel a deeper sense of relaxation as your body comes to associate that space with rest.

Lighting

When setting up your relaxing yoga space, one of the most important steps is perfecting the lighting. Ideally, a space with natural light is best, but a darker corner works well, too, if you set it up properly. To give your space a cozy, calming feel, opt for warmer lighting as opposed to anything fluorescent. Candles work wonders too, allowing you to unwind to the flicker of a warm flame. If you only have cooler bulbs for your lamps, you can drape the lamp to soften the glare and add a cozier ambiance to the space. Some people love to use salt lamps or lanterns to give their space a soft, inviting glow. It's up to you! Humans are sensitive to changes in light, so find the setup that feels right.

Comfort

The final step in setting up your at-home yoga studio is to make your space as comfortable as humanly possible. The steps that you need to take in order to make your practice area as snug and cozy as possible depend entirely on a number of factors. Because the purpose of restorative yoga is full relaxation and rest, your physical comfort is an essential part of the puzzle. While other forms of yoga focus on enduring discomfort and pushing through obstacles, this practice is all about creating the conditions to put your entire being at ease.

When it comes to comfort, heat is one factor you will want to consider. Depending on where your yoga space is located, you may need to have supplies that allow you to warm up or cool down. If you have the choice of several locations in your home, you might want to opt for a room that can be controlled for temperature throughout the year.

Restorative yoga is all about comfort and relaxation, so it's important that your body feels good while you're in this space. This is not easy if you live in a particularly hot or cold climate, so consider the elements when setting up your space. If you're in a drafty room you'll want to fill your room with textiles of varying fabrics and weights; pile in as many quilts, comforters, and rugs as you can to ensure that you always feel cozy. If your space is stuffy, you may want to consider a small fan to create a pleasant breeze.

Finally, think about the flooring in your yoga space. This might seem odd, but it really matters. Because restorative poses are held for longer spans of time than other, more active forms of yoga, you may want to use multiple mats on harder surfaces. Sure, your laminate flooring might feel fine for the first thirty seconds or so, but how will it feel three or four minutes into a pose? In my own practice space, I find it helpful to layer rugs beneath my mat to prevent the hardwood floor from digging into my joints as I sink into each pose. If you live with joint discomfort or chronic pain, you may want to opt for a carpeted space to avoid any surprise sensitivities during your practice. Trust me, the last thing you want to feel during a restful child's pose is a cold ceramic tile digging into your knees!

Props

One of the most important aspects of restorative yoga is the use of props. In restorative yoga, we use objects of varying shapes, textures, weights, and sizes to support the body. It's hard to overstate the importance of props during a restorative yoga flow; in order to fully relax, our muscles need to feel secure and stable in positions that might ordinarily cause strain or tension. Finding appropriate props doesn't need to be a struggle or cost money. Thankfully, most of the props used in this book can be replicated using household items.

Household props you will need:

- Blankets of varying sizes and fabrics
- Towels for rolling and folding
- Sheets for folding and draping
- Pillows in a variety of sizes and densities
- Couch cushions or sturdy pillows
- Washcloths to drape across the eyes
- Chair without wheels for support
- Yoga mat or rug to lie on
- Hot water bottle or heated blanket
- Long scarf or strip of fabric

Additional props you may choose to purchase:

- Yoga bolsters (round and rectangular)
- Pranayama cushion or bolster
- Eye pillow
- Neck pillow
- Yoga blocks
- Yoga strap
- Magic bag
- Weighted blanket

For each pose, I will offer you options for how to support your body with props or household items. Before you begin a flow, ensure that you have everything you need so that you don't have to get up between poses, as this will disrupt your relaxation. Restorative yoga should be a time for you to relax, with as few hassles as possible during transitions.

Clothing

Wear clothing that is comfortable and loose. Some people prefer to wear yoga leggings and sports gear, while others prefer to wear pajamas or loungewear. Choose an outfit that will require very little adjusting and that you won't be distracted by. Avoid anything tight or itchy. Your clothing should not resist stretching or restrict your movement in any way.

Timing

In today's world, time is more precious than ever. It often feels like we don't have enough time in a day to get everything done. From getting enough sleep to making time for family and friends, it can feel like there simply aren't enough minutes to squeeze in things like yoga and meditation. Trust me, I know what it is like to feel stretched thin. I know how it feels to scramble each and every day, desperately trying to stay on top of every aspect of my own hectic schedule. If this sounds familiar to you, I have one piece of advice that will help you build a restorative yoga practice into your hectic routine: start small.

Setting aside fifteen or twenty minutes a day to practice restorative yoga will have an incredible impact on your stress levels and your ability to focus and be present for your current commitments. By taking this time each day, or even a few times a week, you will be giving your body the nurturing care it needs to get you through each challenge life throws at you with confidence and resilience.

In my experience, starting a restorative yoga practice actually made my days feel less, rather than more, busy. Once I began taking the time to really relax, I felt more grounded and more capable when my attention was needed elsewhere. Sure, it's awesome if you can set aside an hour each night to flow through some juicy extended poses. But, if all you have is fifteen minutes, that's enough for now.

How to Use This Book

Each chapter in this book is sectioned by different needs or concerns you might be facing. For example, we have chapters on depression, stress, exhaustion, and more. The chapters are set up in a way that teaches poses specific to the need you have. Some of these poses overlap in other chapters, and I have listed those poses at the beginning of each chapter. This is simply because one pose can offer benefits for multiple issues you may have.

Feel free to jump around the chapters as you look for the poses that will assist you with your problems. You can refer to the end of the book for sequence ideas or tips for how to create your own., or you can simply find one pose at a time that works for you. It's up to you and what your body needs.

If you have any physical limitations such as pregnancy, illness, or something else, be sure to always read the modification section of each pose. And always be sure to check with a doctor before performing any type of new physical exercise.

Now, before you dive into the poses, be sure to read the next chapter which will discuss the very essential foundation of breathing and meditation.

3

BREATHING AND MEDITATION

BEGINNING YOUR PRACTICE: WHY BREATHING & MEDITATION MATTERS

How is your breathing right now? Take a moment to notice. Is it deep? Shallow? Quick? Slow? Notice as your ribs and belly expand and then contract. See if you can inhale a bit deeper and exhale slower.

Our breath is a constant in our lives, tied inextricably to our emotional and physical state. When we are frightened, our breathing becomes rapid and shallow. When we are calm and relaxed, our breathing becomes prolonged, ebbing and flowing like gentle waves against a shoreline. Checking in with our breath is a vital part of connecting with ourselves to become calmer, more resilient, more mindful versions of ourselves. Meditation and pranayama, otherwise known as breathwork, help us to moderate and improve our well-being by forming deeper, more mindful connections between our minds and our bodies.

In this chapter, we will explore the basics of breathwork and meditation. The breath is the foundation of any yoga practice. In traditional Eastern philosophy, pranayama is the fourth limb of the practice of postural, hatha yoga. Simply put, breathwork is the awareness of and the control over our inhalation and exhalation. By manipulating the breath, we can transform our mental and physical states. A strong grasp of breathwork allows us to self-regulate when we are feeling mentally or physically overwrought or out of control. Therefore, pranayama is a natural starting point for learning restorative yoga.

PRANAYAMA FOR RESTORATIVE YOGA

Pranayama is a Sanskrit word that roughly means life force (prana), expansion (ayama), and control (yama). As one of the central pieces of any yoga practice, breathwork is key to unlocking the many incredible benefits of yoga. From relaxation to improved digestion, to improved mental health, pranayama elevates our yoga practice from a purely physical to a holistically beneficial emotional, mental, and spiritual experience.

Before I get into the details of how and when to practice the various styles of breathwork, I want to share my own introductory experience with the practice. When I first started my yoga journey, I was a bit wary of pranayama. This is common for many of us when we first start to practice yoga because we come to the practice thinking about it as a form of exercise. Postures? Great. Movement? Fantastic! But this new breathing thing? I was hesitant at first, to say the least. If you are a driven, fast-paced, practical person, chances are you share in this feeling.

When I first started practicing yoga, I was in high school. I was an angsty, tightly wound kid, up to her neck in friend-ship drama and the daily anxieties that come with the terri-tory of being a teenager. I had a yoga class at the end of each school day, and once my class started, my breathing slowed and I lost myself in the movements and the rhythms of the practice. I had heard teachers and healthcare professionals droning on about the importance of deep breathing and how it helped with anxiety, but I had never actually tried in earnest. After that first class, I was hooked. Something about the combination of slowed breathing and gentle movement transported me out of my brain and into a calmer, more peaceful state.

A key part of what kept me coming back to yoga was the incredible sense of peace I got from breathwork. It became addictive; suddenly, I was incorporating ocean breathing into everything from walking to school each morning to calming myself down during tests. Years later, as an adult practitioner, I am still using pranayama in my daily life, especially when I encounter tantrums from my toddler. I can't overstate what a valuable tool breathwork can be.

Pranayama isn't magic, even if it sure feels like it. It's science. As we discussed in Chapter 1, yoga helps us to regulate our nervous systems. Pranayama, in particular, helps us to slow our breathing, triggering our parasympathetic nervous system to let our bodies know that they are safe to let go of fear, worry, anger, and many other strong emotions. When we practice breathwork, we are communicating with the deepest reaches of our minds to say that it is time to relax. In addition, by breathing deeply we use our diaphragms to massage our digestive tract, encouraging digestion and healthy gut movement. Energetically speaking, pranayama helps us to focus our energy on particular chakras, clearing pathways for our lifeforce to flow freely through us. Regardless of the perspective that resonates most with you, pranayama is a profound and useful tool to support your overall health and well-being.

Preparing for Pranayama Practice

Before you embark on your first pranayama practice, it's important to find a comfortable place to sit. The nicest thing about breathwork is that it can happen anywhere once you have a bit of experience. In the car, at a coffee shop, in the bath—you name the location and it is possible to practice pranayama. Still, if you want to fully commit to a beginner's breathwork practice, it is best to find a location where you can sit comfortably without interruptions or distractions.

Take stock of your posture. Are your shoulders hunched? Are they soft and relaxed? Take a moment and let them release. In order to breathe fully, your ribs must be able to expand and contract with ease, so it is a good idea to scan your torso and hips. Ensure that you feel grounded and that you are sitting tall with an open chest and gentle, soft belly. Before I start my pranayama, I like to do some gentle shoulder circles, letting my shoulders rise up to my ears, then back and down. It can also be more comfortable to sit cross-legged or kneel, depending on your body.

Once you feel ready, try each of the following breathwork styles to find the ones that feel most centering for you. I have my favorites, as I'm sure you will, too. Each of the types of breathwork described in this section can be added to your restorative yoga practice. Simply choose the breath practice that corresponds to the way you want to feel. Some styles are better suited to the beginning or end of a practice, while others are sustainable throughout each pose. Breath is personal. With time, some of these styles will become second nature and blend seamlessly into your practice, as well as your daily life.

Pranayama Practices

1. Balanced Breath

a. Benefits:

This pranayama practice is a simple introductory style that will get you comfortable and grounded to begin your restorative yoga practice. Balanced breath helps you take stock of your body's current state while gently easing you into stillness. This style of breathing helps us to match our inhales and our exhales, bringing harmony and balance to the respiratory system. After just a few rounds of balanced breathing, we can regulate our heartbeats and return our bodies and minds to a resting state. Use this pranayama anytime you feel anxious, overwhelmed, or exhausted. This breath can be helpful during moments of high anxiety or stress in public places as well, as it is simple and subtle. If you are not able to find somewhere to sit, you can practice balanced breathing on the go, simply by counting your breaths from a standing or walking position.

b. Instructions:

Find a comfortable seat and close your eyes. Sit tall, reaching your arms toward the sky with the crown of your head. As you exhale, lower your arms again, slowly to match the speed of your breath. Place your palms face up if you wish to receive energy, or face down if you feel like you need to ground yourself. Inhale slowly to the count of four, counting each number in your mind. When you reach four, pause briefly before counting back down to one as you exhale. Pause briefly again and then repeat the cycle. As you relax into the practice, you may find that you can stretch your breath further into counts of five, six, or seven. Whatever number you choose, make sure that you can breathe easily and that you are not straining. Continue this breath until you feel calm and centered, beginning with a minimum of ten rounds of breath. Feel free to use balanced breathing at the beginning, middle, or end of your restorative yoga practice.

2. Apa Japa Breath

a. Benefits:

The benefits of this form of pranayama include increased focus, mental clarity, and gentle relaxation. Apa Japa Breath is a meditative form of breathwork, in which you focus on your own breathing patterns and resist the temptation to interfere with your body's natural pacing and rhythm. This style of breathwork enhances your self-awareness and grounds you firmly in the present moment by preventing your mind from wandering. Use this practice when you want to feel more in touch with your body and your emotions. Apa Japa can be helpful when you are feeling disoriented, frustrated, or upset as it forces you to turn inward and away from the chaotic external world. It can also be a perfect starting point for any restorative yoga practice.

b. Instructions:

Find a comfortable seat and close your eyes. Bring your awareness to your chest, ribs, and belly. You may choose to place one hand on your chest and one on your abdomen. Notice your body expand and contract with each inhale and exhale. Resist the urge to judge or alter your breath. Simply observe each rise and fall, focusing on the breath as is, natural and gentle. Continue to observe your breathing until you feel calm and ready to continue your practice in a state of physical and mental stillness. This could take anywhere from ten to fifteen breath cycles.

3. Sitkari Breath

a. Benefits:

Sitkari pranayama is a calming breath that helps to regulate your nervous system. Practicing Sitkari Breath can reduce anxiety and help with insomnia.

While using this breath practice, draw your attention to your crown chakra to access deeper levels of clarity and focus. While it may seem unusual that this breath-work style can both increase your ability to focus and prepare your mind for sleep, it is actually capable of doing both. Regardless of whether you want to wind down or focus, Sitkari pranayama clears your mind in preparation for any challenge. Use Sitkari pranayama when you want to alleviate stress, calm your nerves, or enhance your focus.

b. Instructions:

Sit in a comfortable position, with your shoulders relaxed and your spine long. Raise your chin slightly so that your jaw is parallel with the floor. Bring your tongue to touch the back of your lower teeth and hold it flat against the bottom of your mouth. Open your mouth slightly and inhale slowly, noticing the air as it travels across your tongue to the back of your throat. When you finish inhaling, close your lips. Exhale through your nose, slowly. Part your lips and begin the process a second time. Continue the cycle for a minimum of ten breaths.

4. Three-Part Breath

a. Benefits:

Three-Part Breath is a simple, rhythmic pranayama that helps you access your full lung capacity. This style has a variety of benefits, from improving digestion to increasing energy and restoring calm. The soothing, structured pattern of this breathwork practice is perfect for calming the mind and can be used to combat depression, anxiety, and trauma. Use this pranayama when you need to refocus your energy or shift your awareness away from the struggles of your daily life. Lose yourself in the rhythm of Three-Part Breath and emerge at the end of the practice feeling lighter and clearer.

b. Instructions:

This breath can be practiced lying down or from a seated position. Make yourself comfortable and exhale as you release any tension from your core. Allow your shoulders to drop and your jaw to soften. Bring one hand to your chest and the other to your belly. Inhale into your chest, feeling your hand rise slightly as your lungs expand. When you feel that you have inhaled to approximately one-quarter of your lung capacity, pause, retaining the air. Then, inhale into your belly, drawing in additional air until your lungs are at capacity and you feel both your belly and your chest fully expanded. Pause here, noticing the sensations, before exhaling slowly until you have expelled all of the air from your lungs. Pause one last time before beginning the cycle again. As you inhale, find a natural rhythm, ensuring that your exhale is always as long, if not longer, than your two-part inhale. Move through at least ten breath cycles, until you feel ready to move on to the next part of your practice.

5. Ujjayi Breath

a. Benefits:

Ujjayi Breath is one of the most popular pranayama styles in all of yoga. This breath practice is very popular in yoga studios and lends itself well to moving practices, such as vinyasa and ashtanga yoga. Also known as Ocean Breath, Ujjayi Breath is a noisier pranayama style that helps you remain physically and mentally focused on your breath throughout your practice. This breath can be used when you want to create a more intentional breath, warm up the body after a long sleep, or refocus your wandering mind. Use this breath style to immerse yourself in a fully present warm-up flow and to clear your mind as you begin to move toward longer restorative poses.

b. Instructions:

Ujjayi Breath can be practiced in stillness or in motion. In this pranayama, you will inhale through your nose and exhale through your mouth. Always begin in stillness, ideally in a seated position or lying on your back. Use your soft palate and tongue to restrict the airflow as it moves through your nose and throat. The restriction should be enough that you can hear the air as it moves. The sound this restriction creates is like the hum of the ocean as waves crash and recede against a shoreline. As you inhale, imagine that you are trying to snore, but only loud enough that it is audible for you and perhaps another person if they were in the same room. As you exhale through your nose, make the breath audible again, like a forceful sigh. Breathe only through your nose, slowly, audibly, and deliberately. Once you have mastered this rhythm, you can begin to move. Your breath should remain audible throughout your practice as you focus on your Ujjayi Breath alongside each pose. If you are moving between poses, do so on exhalations. Follow the rhythm of this breath in the more active portion of your practice. When you are ready to move into the relaxation phase of your restorative practice, release this breath.

6. Alternate Nostril Breath

a. Benefits:

Alternate Nostril Breathing is a form of pranayama that requires mindful attention and coordination. It is useful for centering and balancing the mind while providing a gentle, cognitive challenge. The benefits of this pranayama practice include lowering your heart rate, improving your lung capacity, and deep relaxation. Use this breath at the beginning and the end of your practice, or when you are feeling like you need a quick re-centering throughout the day.

b. Instructions:

Find a comfortable seated position. Sit tall, with your shoulders relaxed and your chest open. Place your left hand on your leg and bring your right hand to the top of your nose. Allow your left nostril to remain open while using your fingers to close your right nostril. Inhale through the left nostril, filling your lungs with air. Pinch both nostrils closed as you retain the air and pause here. Open the right nostril to exhale as you keep the left closed. When you have exhaled fully, pause before inhaling now through the right nostril. Pause at the end of your inhale before closing the right nostril, opening the left, and exhaling. Repeat this process from the beginning, alternating between nostrils. Continue this pranayama for at least eight breath cycles.

MEDITATION FOR RESTORATIVE YOGA

Meditation is a powerful tool to add to your yoga practice. There are many kinds of meditation, each with specific aims and philosophies. In this book, we will mainly talk about mindfulness meditation. This is a simple form of meditation that is easy and accessible, regardless of your experience level.

On its own, meditation has been shown to have a wide variety of benefits. From reduced stress and anxiety to improved self-esteem and productivity, the effects of this practice are pretty remarkable. While it can seem scary and intimidating at first, mindfulness meditation is actually very simple. All you need to do is close your eyes, notice your thoughts, and accept them without judgment. Pretty easy, right?

In this section, we will go over several visualizations and meditations that you can use at the beginning of your practice before you begin your warm-up. Starting your restorative yoga practice with meditation is a great way to calm your mind and prepare you for a slow, relaxing series of poses. By meditating prior to your warm-up, you can ensure that you start your practice wholly present and mindful. Visualizations, on the other hand, can be helpful to pair with your meditation and pranayama practice. When you use a visualization, you focus your mental energy. This is helpful if you have a particularly wandering mind.

1. Visualizations

a. Rainstorm:

> This visualization is the perfect antidote to a stressful day. Use it when you are feeling frustrated, over-whelmed, or overworked. Take a comfortable seat and close your eyes. Imagine yourself in a natural location; picture somewhere far from the busy world you normally inhabit. Look up to see the sky, filled with heavy clouds. Inside those clouds is a brewing storm. This storm isn't just filled with rain and thunder; this storm is made of every stress in your life: every disap-pointment, every problem, every frustration is rumbling somewhere deep inside these grey clouds. Take a deep inhale and watch the rain begin to fall. Slowly at first, and then faster, and heavier, until the whole world around you is consumed by thick sheets of falling rain. Listen to the sound as you let the water wash over you, blanketing the earth, beating the ground, the trees, every inch of your skin. Look up as you breathe, watching the storm. Take a deep breath in and exhale as you raise your arms up, fully letting go of any control. Now, begin to notice the rain growing softer. With every breath, the rain is slowing,

becoming lighter. Take one more breath in and as you exhale, watch the clouds begin to open. Watch as beams of light break through the darkness and the sky opens. Listen as birds chirp, and wind blows through the leaves of trees. Feel the warm sunlight on your skin. Take a deep breath here, noticing the weight that has lifted.

b. Waves:

This is a breathing visualization, best used for relaxation and mindful pranayama. Find a comfortable seat and close your eyes. Picture yourself seated on a rock overlooking the sea. With every inhale, watch the waves recede, pulling back from the shoreline. Pause, watching the water swell. Exhale as you watch the waves rush forward, crashing along the shore. Pace your breathing with the ebb and flow of the tides, letting yourself let go. If it feels good, sway to the natural rhythm of the ocean.

c. Sphere:

This is a visualization that works well with a variety of pranayama styles. Use it when you want to turn inward and focus on your breath. In a comfortable, seated position, close your eyes and relax your shoulders, forehead, and jaw. Imagine a sphere floating in space. As you inhale, it expands, growing larger as it fills with breath. On the exhale, it shrinks as you expel air until it returns to its original size. Try to breathe continuously, so that the sphere expands and contracts in one smooth, slow motion. If you want to make this visualization more physical, you can hold your hands out in front of you as if you are holding the sphere. Move your hands as it expands on the inhale, and shrinks on the exhale. Follow this cycle for as long as you need.

2. Meditations

a. Body Scan:

This meditation can be done seated or lying down. Close your eyes and bring your awareness to your toes, simply noticing them. Draw your awareness upward, noticing sensations in the soles of your feet and your ankles. Pause here. Move again, traveling up to notice your calves and shins. Notice how they feel right now, without judgment. Move your awareness to the front and back of your knees. Next, your thighs, hips, glutes, and pelvis. Pause here, bringing your awareness to any sensations you might be feeling right now. Next, focus your awareness on your abdomen, scanning your tailbone, lower back, and belly. Travel up again, moving your awareness to your ribs and middle back. Next, move upward again, now noticing your chest, sternum, and shoulder blades. Scan them without judgment before shifting your awareness to your shoulders, upper arms, elbows, wrists, palms, and fingertips. Pause here. Move now to notice your throat, your neck, and your ears. Bring your awareness to your lower jaw, noticing any sensations or tension here. Travel now to your lips, your cheeks, your temples, your eyes, your scalp. Pause here, bringing your full awareness next to your forehead. Let it rest here momentarily before focusing finally on the crown of your head. When you are ready, open your eyes.

b. Progressive Muscle Relaxation:

This meditation is very similar to a body scan and follows the same pattern as above. In a body scan, you simply notice each part of the body, while this meditation takes it one step further. As you scan each part of your body, focus on relaxing any tension and softening the muscles fully. This meditation can be used before bedtime or in corpse pose to combat fatigue, insomnia, and anxiety.

c. Gratitude:

This gratitude meditation is a simple daily practice to combat emotional and mental health challenges such as depression, anxiety, and/or grief. In this meditation, you focus on breathing calmly while picturing the people, places, and things that you are grateful for in your life. You can try to think of multiple sources of gratitude or meditate on one simple aspect of your life that you are grateful for. The idea is to try to push your feelings of gratitude out into the world, allowing the feelings to wash over you as you sit in silence.

d. Compassion:

Compassion is a powerful force that not only helps us to treat others with kindness but ourselves as well. For this meditation, select one person, situation, or problem in your life that is causing you to feel negative emotions or presenting obstacles in your life. This will be your focal point for the meditation practice. As you breathe, imagine that you are exhaling love, forgiveness, and patience toward this focal point, enveloping them in positive feelings. Inhale strength, resilience, and peacefulness, while exhaling compassion. As you meditate, notice your emotions toward this focal point begin to shift, and the weight or tension you are carrying begin to lift away, leaving you more centered and less frustrated.

PUTTING THE PIECES TOGETHER

When you are ready to begin your restorative yoga practice, there are several ways to sequence pranayama, meditation, and poses. My personal favorite is the following structure:

1. Pranayama
2. Meditation
3. Warm-Up
4. Pose Flow
5. Pranayama

I enjoy bookending my practice with the same pranayama, returning to the breath at the end of my practice as a gentle check-in before ending my practice. You may find a structure that speaks to you more, so play around with your practice until you find an order that feels right. It's important, though, to ensure that you begin with pranayama and a warm-up before getting into your main poses. This helps you mentally and physically prepare for the practice. Warm-ups, in particular, are critically important. In the next chapter, I will give you a few examples to use and explain how to organize your warm-up.

4

WARMING UP

Picture yourself on a busy freeway. Cars are racing by as you weave through traffic, your mind constantly aware of a handful of variables. How close is the car in front of you? How fast should you be going? Will you be on time? Imagine the sound of horns honking, radios blaring. Now, picture yourself as you exit the freeway onto the off-ramp; imagine the slow, gentle curve of the road as it bends, easing your car back down to a manageable speed before you rejoin the less frantic world of regular traffic. Could you simply turn right off of a busy freeway and rejoin regular city traffic without an off-ramp? The idea feels ridiculous, not to mention unsafe.

Our lives, like busy freeways, require us to be on our toes, moving at warp speed. In order to juggle the demands of daily life, we are always in motion, either mentally, physically, or both. Just like our vehicles need off-ramps to slow down, our bodies need warm-ups to help us slow down as we enter a yoga practice. One of the biggest reasons that newcomers to restorative yoga struggle is that they have a difficult time "switching off" after a busy day. Sitting still for an extended period of time can be a serious challenge for those of us with hectic or stressful lives. In fact, doing so can feel jarring without a proper warm-up because our bodies need the chance to slow down and ease into a restorative practice.

Like other forms of physical activity, restorative yoga requires an effective warm-up. Unlike those for more strenuous workouts or more active yoga styles, restorative warm-ups actually help us to slow down, rather than speed up. In this chapter, you will learn a comprehensive warm-up to ease you out of your busy life and into your relaxation practice.

WARM-UP FLOWS

Each of these flows is designed to be used in your warm-up. Feel free to organize your own warm-up using whichever flows speak to you and feel good. The purpose of this section is simply to provide you with a toolkit to design your own warm-ups. Ideally, try to combine three to four of these flows in order to ease yourself into each of your restorative yoga practices.

The eight warm-up flows we will explore in this chapter are:

1. Cat and Cow Flow
2. Shoulder Circles Flow
3. Low Back Massage Flow
4. Eagle Arms Flow
5. Knee-to-Chest Flow (also seen in Chapters 6 & 7; also known as Wind-Relieving Pose)
6. Low Lunge to Forward Fold Flow
7. Flowing Seated Twists
8. Seated Side Stretch Flow

The only props you will require for these warm-up flows are a yoga mat, a small cushion or pillow, and a yoga block or thick hardcover book.

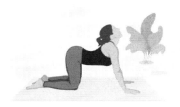 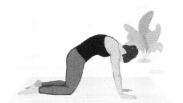

1. Cat and Cow Flow

a. Targets:

This basic warm-up flow wakes up your entire core as you bring gentle movement to your spine. Cat and cow are the perfect poses to work between when you are feeling stiff, tired, or unbalanced. As you move through these poses, you will likely feel an increased awareness of your heart and throat chakras. Cat and cow poses are considered standard, essential poses for a reason; nothing beats the feeling of catharsis and release that comes with this simple flow.

b. Instructions:

Come to a table-top position on your mat, on all
fours. Place your hands beneath your shoulders and
press into the mat with wide fingertips. Ensure that
your knees are directly beneath your hips and that
your toes are either gently tucked or laying flat on the
mat. Play around with your shoulder blades for a
moment until you find a neutral position where your
chest feels open and your shoulders feel engaged. As
you inhale, drop your belly to the mat, expanding
your torso with your breath. Tilt your pelvis back and
up as you shine your chest to the sky and bring your
gaze to follow. Pause here momentarily before
exhaling and rounding through the spine, bringing
your gaze toward your knees and pushing into the
floor with your hands. Tuck your tailbone and round
through your back, creating an arch along your spine
from the back of your head to your glutes. When you
are ready to inhale again, repeat this flow, moving
from cat to cow with each inhale and exhale, allowing
your breath to guide and pace the movement. Move as
slowly and deliberately as you are able. If you choose
to pair this movement with pranayama practice, you
might choose to use a Balanced or Ujjayi Breath. Both
are appropriate styles for this flow and will complement the movements for a moving meditation.

c. Modifications:

If you have any wrist or ankle pain, this pose is easily modified to create space and support for your joints. For knee pain, place a folded blanket, cushion, or towel beneath your knees. For your wrists, you can use a folded blanket or pillows beneath your hands. Some people find it helpful to make fists and rest on their knuckles to avoid putting weight onto the wrists altogether. If you are pregnant, you may choose to do this flow standing with your arms placed on a chair or low table so that your torso is on an incline rather than fully parallel to the ground. Tucking or untucking the toes is a matter of preference, so play around with the pose before you begin to ensure you feel stable and comfortable.

d. Duration:

Guide yourself through this flow for a minimum of 10 breath cycles.

2. Shoulder Circles Flow

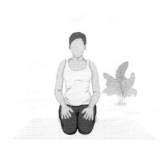 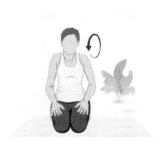

a. Targets:

This flow helps to mobilize your shoulders. It brings awareness to the head, neck, and shoulders, where many of us hold tension from stress throughout the day. By working this flow into your practice, you will invite this part of your upper body to soften and open. Through this flow, you will have opportunities to open your solar plexus, heart, and throat chakras.

b. Instructions:

Find a comfortable seat, ideally in a kneeling position. If this isn't accessible for you, you can sit with your legs crossed or in a butterfly position with the soles of your feet pressed together and your knees wide. Sit tall and imagine a string pulling the crown of your head up to the sky. It may feel good to move the flesh of your glutes out from under you so that your hips are more grounded. Place your palms on your thighs and lower your gaze. Take a moment to breathe before drawing your shoulders up toward your ears on your first inhale of the flow. Next, let them drift back and then down, away from your ears as you exhale. Continue this pattern in this direction before switching to reverse the flow.

c. Modifications:

If you find it challenging to sit on the floor, this flow can be performed in a chair or in a standing position. Another way to support this pose is to sit on a cushion or pillow so that your hips are elevated.

d. Duration:

Continue this flow for a minimum of 6 breath cycles in each direction.

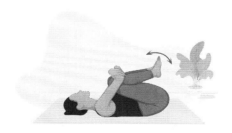

3. Low Back Massage Flow

a. Targets:

This flow is a fabulous tool for loosening up your hips, glutes, and lower back using only your body weight and a bit of momentum. Use this flow when you're experiencing any kind of lower back pain, from cramps to arthritis to post-workout aches.

b. Instructions:

Lie on your back. Bring your knees toward your chest and hold them close to your torso. Begin to rock from side to side, mindfully massaging your lower back and hips with the floor. Move slowly and find the points of most tension, releasing the muscles gently. Notice a slight stretch through your shoulder blades as you hold your legs firmly.

c. Modifications:

If you are pregnant or have limited mobility, you may want to use a yoga strap to hold your legs. Either tie the strap around your back and loop it behind your knees or hold it with your hands. If you don't have a yoga strap, a scarf will work well, too.

d. Duration:

Roll from side to side at least 10 times, breathing mindfully.

4. Eagle Arms Flow

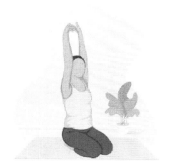 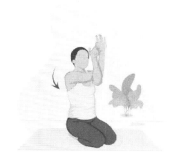

a. Targets:

This warm-up flow targets your upper back and shoulders while providing a light cognitive challenge for your mind. This flow can feel complex at first but becomes second nature once you get the hang of it. During this flow, focus on breathing into the space between your shoulder blades as you expand on each inhale, creating space through your chest and heart chakra.

b. Instructions:

Find a comfortable seat, ideally in a kneeling or cross-legged position. Reach your arms up overhead. Swing both arms down and forward, sweeping one arm under the other so that both elbows are bent, tucked together snuggly, with your forearms vertical. Wrap your wrists and hands together, pointing your fingertips toward the ceiling. Inhale and expand your rib cage out and back, stretching the space between your shoulder blades and along your outer arms. Exhale and unwind your arms, reaching overhead. Repeat the process with the other arm underneath now. Continue to repeat this process, moving with your breath.

c. Modifications:

If your shoulders are tight or you have a larger chest, you may choose to modify this flow. One way to do so is to bring your arms out to the sides and wrap them around your body, giving yourself a tight hug. This will give you a similar stretch without the added complication of the arm positioning described above. Open your arms to inhale, and then close them, hugging yourself tight, with each exhale. Both versions of this flow will target the upper back and shoulders, with some very minor differences.

d. Duration:

Continue this flow for a minimum of 10 breath cycles before moving on.

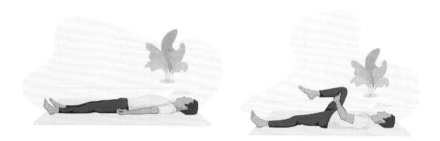

5. Knee-to-Chest Flow

a. Targets:

This simple flow targets your hips, abdomen, legs, and back through gentle, linear movements. As you move through this part of your warm-up, focus your attention on grounding yourself through the floor. This flow wakes up your sacral and crown chakras as you root these two points to your mat, moving from the firm foundation of your savasana.

b. Instructions:

Lie on your back, adjusting your shoulders and hips into a comfortable neutral position. Point your toes long and reach tall through the crown of your head, stretching your entire body along the floor. Take a breath in and as you exhale, lift your left leg up off the floor, bending at the knee. Hold your left leg to your chest, feeling a gentle stretch along your lower back, glutes, and hamstrings. Inhale here and exhale, lowering your leg back down to the floor. Repeat this process on the other side, moving to the rhythm of your breath as you go.

c. Modifications:

If you want a calf stretch, you can keep your legs straight and flex your toes as you move through this flow. This will allow you to feel a stretch through the backs of your legs but may require more core work.

d. Duration:

Move through this flow for a minimum of 6 breath cycles, using the sensations in your body as a guide. If you feel like this flow is serving your body, add additional cycles.

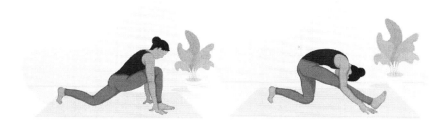

6. Low Lunge to Forward Fold Flow

a. Targets:

This flow targets the muscles throughout your legs, including your glutes, hamstrings, hip flexors, calves, quads, and feet. The fluid motions work to open up your muscles and release any tension, physical or emotional, that you have accumulated throughout the day. We often hold a lot of emotion in our hips, so it is normal to feel waves of negative emotions emerge as you move through this flow. You may find an opening in your throat chakra, so this pose pairs well with Ujjayi Breath as this pranayama engages this area.

b. Instructions:

Find a kneeling position on your mat, standing tall on your knees with your shins and feet resting on the floor. Bring one knee up and forward as you plant that foot firmly on the mat so that you are in a half-kneeling position. Inhaling, tilt your pelvis forward before moving your hips forward toward your raised knee, planting your fingers on the ground on either side of your leg. Feel the stretch through the front of your other leg and hip flexor. As you exhale, send your hips back toward your feet and bow forward, bringing your torso toward your knee. Straighten that front leg for a deeper stretch as you bow. On the inhale, move forward again, continuing the flow. Repeat this cycle on one leg before moving on to the other side to balance the stretch and repeat the process again.

c. Modifications:

You may find it more comfortable to place a cushion, pillow, towel, or blanket beneath your grounded knee for support. In addition, be mindful of your knee by keeping a slight bend in each leg as it straightens.

d. Duration:

Flow through this motion for 5 breath cycles per side, ensuring that you complete the same number of flows on each side.

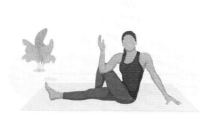 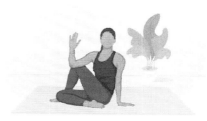

7. Flowing Seated Twists

a. Targets:

This dynamic flow targets your spine, upper back, lower back, hips, legs, and core for a gentle, full-body stretch. The twisting nature of this flow aids in digestion and helps to bring your body's attention to your internal organs as they gently compress with each twist. This flow is a nice go-to when you are experiencing indigestion or constipation. During this sequence, focus your mind on your third eye chakra, expanding your awareness as you reach with each stretch.

b. Instructions:

Sit tall on your mat with your legs long in front of you. Bring one foot to the outside of your opposite knee, planting it firmly on the floor. Bend your opposite arm, hooking the elbow on the inside of your bent knee, bracing as you twist. Keep your shoulders relaxed as you sit tall, twisting, your gaze moving over your shoulder as you corkscrew out of your seat. If it feels good, bend your outstretched knee, placing the foot next to your hip. Otherwise, keep your leg outstretched. Unwind slowly and carefully on an inhale, mindfully placing your leg back to the floor. Switch sides, moving through the twist in the opposite direction now. Do not force the twist if you feel tense through the spine. Flexibility will come with time and patience.

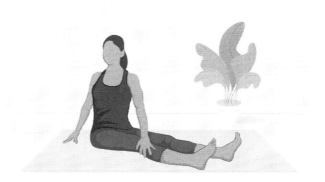

c. Modifications:

There are many ways to modify this pose. You may find it uncomfortable to sit on the floor without support. In this case, use a cushion to elevate your hips and take the pressure off of your leg muscles. Alternatively, if you have limited mobility, you may want to use a strap to hold your knee close to your torso or grip your leg differently. These modifications are all possible and easy to adjust as you move through the flow. If you are pregnant or in a larger body, you can leave both legs long on the floor and twist. In this modification, place your hands on the floor and the outer side of your thigh for support and stability.

d. Duration:

Work through this flow for a minimum of 6 breath cycles, or for however long feels right for your body today.

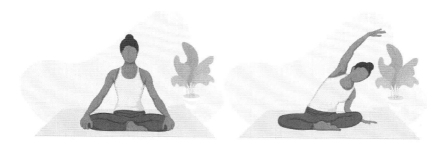

8. Seated Side Stretch Flow

a. Targets:

This flow addresses the muscles along the side of your body, including your core, hips, and arms. As you move through this flow, notice as these muscles activate and begin to open. In my experience, this flow is a wonderful one to integrate into a morning routine as it helps to wake up your entire upper body.

b. Instructions:

Find a comfortable seated position, either with butterfly legs or crossed legs. Ensure that your hips are rooted firmly to the ground before inhaling and reaching one arm up in a sweeping arc. Stretch the length of that side of your body as you reach your arm up and over your head. As you exhale, lower your arm back down in a reverse motion, coming back to a neutral position. Repeat on the other side, flowing with your breath. Continue this cycle.

c. Modifications:

If you are uncomfortable sitting directly on the floor, this flow can be done from a cushion or even a chair. Ensure that your hips stay touching the floor as you move. If one side pops up, reduce the movement a bit.

d. Duration:

Continue this flow for at least 10 breath cycles, ensuring equal numbers of stretches on each side.

5

BACK PAIN

Parenthood comes with a variety of new struggles and challenges. When my first child was born, I was over the moon, like any new mother. Chasing my little one around the house as she grew, I began to experience new aches and pains. Constant lifting, squatting, bending, and bouncing, combined with a total lack of regular sleep, meant that my body was overworked and running on fumes. By my daughter's first birthday, I had begun to experience the type of lower back pain I had grown up hearing women in my family sigh about. No matter what I did, the dull, throbbing ache across my tailbone and hips returned each day with what felt like increasing strength.

Anyone who has experienced back pain knows how overwhelming it can be. Back pain afflicts people from all walks of life; regardless of whether young or old, rich or poor, you are just as likely to experience soreness along your spine and upper hips. Back pain makes people irritable, tired, and withdrawn when it goes untreated. Because our bodies rely on regular, consistent rest to heal and rebuild from our injuries, back pain can feel like a never-ending loop as it keeps us up at night, denying us the sleep we so desperately need to keep it at bay. Thankfully, this doesn't have to be the case! Restorative yoga is an incredible way to heal your sore muscles and put an end to the cycle of back pain.

WHAT CAUSES BACK PAIN?

When talking about back pain, it is important to remember that our spines play a central and vital role in our overall health. Energetically and physically, our backs are the infor-mation superhighway through our bodies, sending vital energy and messages to every inch of our anatomy. If you are experiencing new, painful sensations, it is always best to consult with a doctor to make sure your back pain isn't being caused by something out of the ordinary, like a disc injury or a pinched nerve. This is always best handled first by either medical experts or bodywork practitioners.

Everyday back pain is caused by a variety of factors, both physical and emotional. Repetitive motions, such as bending or lifting, can lead to strain that can leave you feeling sore and overworked. Working at a desk can also contribute to your back pain, especially when you tend to work on a computer or spend time hunched over reading.

On the other hand, chronic back pain can also come from stress, burnout, and trauma. Our bodies use pain as a way to signal danger. When we cut ourselves, our nerves send messages to our brains that something is wrong and we experience those messages as a sharp pain. Sometimes, when we have been put in situations that feel overwhelmingly threatening or stressful, our minds begin to confuse regular stress with immediate danger. This can lead to chronic, stress-based pain in areas like the lower back, shoulders, and hips. Just because one type of pain is from a physical injury and the other is from stress does not mean one is any less real than the other. Pain is pain.

Whether your back pain is due to a specific lifting injury, or ongoing, chronic exhaustion, restorative yoga can help you regain your sense of comfort and foster resilience in your body.

HOW RESTORATIVE YOGA HELPS

Restorative yoga has had a huge impact on my back pain—far more of an impact, in fact, than any hot water bottle or anti-inflammatory ever did. The reasons behind my experience are really fascinating, too. As we have already discussed, restorative yoga is all about relaxation and healing. Whether your back pain is caused by physical, mental, or emotional issues, restorative yoga gives your body the deep, mindful rest it needs to begin the healing process. By activating your parasympathetic nervous system, a regular restorative practice lets your body know that it is safe to repair itself and address areas of discomfort. Intentional, supported rest, combined with gentle stretching, gives your back the nurturing kindness it so badly needs.

RESTORATIVE POSES FOR BACK PAIN

In this section, you will learn about the following poses and their specific benefits for relieving back pain. Each pose comes with modifications to suit your needs and preferences.

1. Supine Figure Four
2. Thread the Needle
3. Supported Bridge (similar variations also seen in Chapters 6 & 10)
4. Supported Backbend (similar variation also seen in Chapter 10)
5. Savasana with Legs on Chair
6. Child's Pose (similar variations also seen in Chapters 7 & 9)
7. Melting Heart Pose (also seen in Chapter 6)
8. Legs up the Wall (similar variations also seen in Chapters 8, 9 & 10)

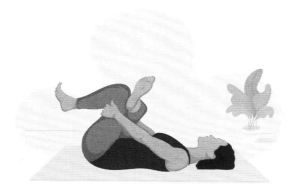

1. Supine Figure Four

a. Benefits:

Supine figure four is a gentle, easily modified pose that offers targeted relief to the hips and lower back. Each side of the pose also provides elevation for your legs and feet. This supports the body in draining lymphatic fluid, gently alleviates pressure on the circulatory system, and offers your tired feet some time to rest after a long day. Hip-opening poses are particularly beneficial for lower back pain, as we often hold tension in our hips that impacts our back muscles. Supine figure four is a more accessible hip-opener for people in larger bodies, too, as it allows space for easy adjustments depending on your needs. This pose is also beneficial for women suffering from low back pain related to menstrual cramping, as it gently massages the mid-back and creates space across the low back and hips.

b. Duration:

Hold this pose for 3 to 6 minutes per side.

c. Props:

- Pillows or bolsters
- Blankets
- Yoga strap or scarf
- Chair or stool

d. Instructions:

Begin by lying down on a comfortable, flat surface. Place the soles of your feet on the mat comfortably close to your glutes. You may choose to elevate your hips slightly on a soft pillow or a folded blanket. Cross one leg to bring your ankle to rest on the top of the opposite thigh, creating a triangle of space between your legs. You may choose to stack bolsters or pillows beneath your knees and thighs to support this pose. To gently stretch your hips, loop your hands around the thigh of your planted leg. If it feels good, drape a blanket or pillow across your abdomen. Be sure to remain passive in this pose. The focus should remain on your breath, gently opening your hip, and relaxing into the pose.

e. Modifications:

If you find this pose uncomfortable for any reason, there are several modifications you can try. If you want to open your hips but find it strenuous to maintain a hold on your thigh, you may choose to lift your planted leg onto a chair to increase the passive stretch through your hip. This added support can feel more grounding, especially when you add a comfortable pillow or blanket to the seat of the chair. Another option for those with limited mobility is to use a yoga strap or scarf to gently bring your thigh toward you. If the strap is long enough, you can even tie a simple knot to loop the strap around your legs and low back. This option allows you to release your arms to the sides for even more relaxation.

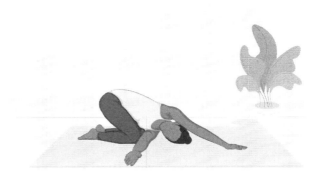

2. Thread the Needle

a. Benefits:

Thread the needle is a simple pose that stretches the upper back and shoulders while increasing spinal mobility. By twisting through the upper spine, this pose stretches between your shoulder blades to alleviate the tension that often builds throughout the course of a busy day. While this pose is often used in more active forms of yoga as a deep stretch, thread the needle in restorative yoga is a gentler, less strenuous variation.

b. Duration:

Hold this pose for 3 to 6 minutes per side.

c. Props:

- Comfortable mat, towel, or rug
- Folded blanket or towel
- Pillows or cushions for stacking

d. Instructions

This pose can easily be done with or without props, depending on your level of flexibility. If you find that this pose feels intense for your body, props are recommended. Kneel on your mat. Stack several pillows or cushions directly in front of your knees. Drape your abdomen and chest over these props. Ensure that the pile is high enough to meet your belly and chest as they come to rest. Lift your right arm overhead before bringing it under your left arm, palm up and arm outstretched along the mat. Bring your weight onto your legs, torso, and the backside of your right shoulder. Place your left arm either on top of your right or along your mat. This twist should be gentle but noticeable. Relax into the support of the props and the mat. When you are finished, repeat on the other side.

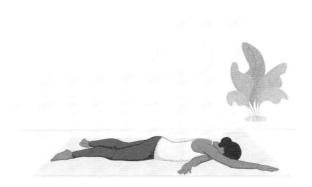

e. Modifications:

If you are in a larger body or have sensitive joints, you may want to increase the cushioning beneath your knees for this pose. If it feels good, you may also prefer a wider stance between your knees. Play around with your leg placement until you find a position that is sustainable for the duration of the pose on both sides. Another relaxing alternative is to lie down fully on the mat while you stretch.

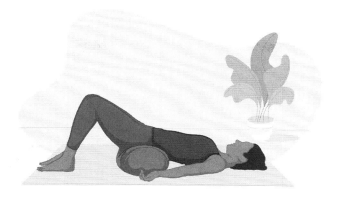

3. Supported Bridge

a. Benefits:

Supported bridge is a gentle and effective pose for coping with back pain. This pose offers both immediate relief and preventative, long-term care for your lower back in particular. When done carefully, this pose offers your lower and mid-back muscles the chance to release, while giving your hip flexors and abdomen a soft opening stretch. Many people find that the supported elevation of this pose also alleviates pressure on the hips and back.

b. Duration:

Hold this pose for 5 to 15 minutes.

c. Props:

- Pillows or cushions
- Bolster or a rolled blanket
- Yoga block or stacked books

d. Instructions:

Lie down on your back on a comfortable surface, such as a thick mat, rug, or blanket. Bend your knees and place your heels as close to your glutes as is comfortable for you. Ideally, you want your knees to be pointing upward toward the ceiling and for your feet to be approximately hip-width apart. Do what feels right for your body in terms of spacing. Next, slowly peel your tailbone off the floor, raising your hips to the sky one vertebra at a time. Place whatever props you have available under your hips and lower back to support your hips, ensuring that they are dense enough to keep your lower body lifted. Be mindful of your tailbone and try to keep your pubic bone tucked to create space along the lower part of your spine and across your hips. Stack your props to a height that feels comfortable and supportive. Close your eyes and relax into the pose as you breathe.

e. Modifications:

In this pose, you may find that you want more cushioning beneath your back to help you fully relax. Some people find it helpful to tie a strap or scarf around their knees so that they don't have to engage their inner thighs in this pose. If you find yourself straining in any way, consider this modification. Depending on your comfort levels, you might opt to use a stack of books or a yoga block beneath your hips. For some people, this doesn't feel as comfortable. Notice what feels best for your body and make the necessary adjustments at the beginning to ensure the pose feels good as you sink into a relaxed state.

4. Supported Backbend

a. Benefits:

Supported backbend works wonders for upper and mid-back pain. This simple, customizable pose offers tension release and helps relieve stiffness through the back and shoulders. One of the reasons that the supported backbend is so popular amongst restorative yogis is because it is incredibly simple and can be done using a wide variety of available household items instead of props. Regardless of which part of your spine you wish to target, this pose can help you find relief.

b. Duration:

Hold this pose for 2 to 10 minutes.

c. Props:

- Bolster or rolled towel
- Pillows or folded blankets
- Blanket or towel

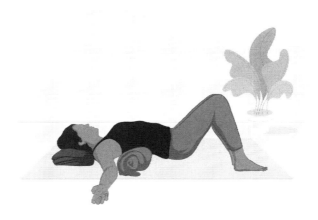

d. Instructions:

Lie on your back. Slowly press up to sit with your legs
outstretched. Behind you, place a thick pillow, bolster,
or rolled towel parallel to the short end of your mat.
Depending on where you want to feel the stretch,
move the prop up or down to a location along your
spine. Then, slowly lower yourself back onto the mat.

Let your muscles relax as you sink into the mat. Remain in this pose for 2 to 3 minutes. If you feel like extending this pose, move the props to a new location along your spine after 3 minutes and repeat the process.

e. Modifications

When setting up this pose, it is important to consider the size of the rolled towel, bolster, or pillow before you lie down. The larger the size, the more intense the stretch will feel. If it helps you to feel more grounded, drape a blanket or towel across your torso as you close your eyes.

5. Savasana with Legs on a Chair

a. Benefits:

This modified version of savasana offers all the calming benefits of the relaxing classic without any of the lower back pressure. By including a chair in this pose, you can simultaneously relax while gently elongating the back body, including your hamstrings, glutes, and back. Savasana itself is a wonderful pose for grounding, offering a chance to check in with your breath and practice mindful belly breathing. This variation forces your spine to root firmly into the floor, offering some healing pressure to your lower back in particular. Elevating the legs also gives your entire body a chance to recalibrate from a long day of standing.

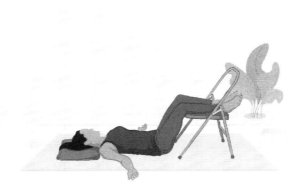

b. Duration:

Hold this pose for 3 to 6 minutes, depending on how long you have been on your feet. Extending this pose is a great way to finish your practice before a final savasana, so pick the duration that fits your practice.

c. Props:

- Chair, coffee table, couch, or ottoman
- Blanket or soft pillow
- Additional blanket or towel

d. Instructions:

Bring a chair, small table, or ottoman onto your mat. If you do not have one of these handy, a couch will work well too. Place a soft blanket or pillow on top if the surface is not cushioned already. Situate yourself so that the chair or other furniture item is snug to your glutes. Roll onto your back, gently swinging your legs onto the elevated surface. Notice the floor pressing into your spine and tilt your hips to ground your lower back. From here, place your palms onto your belly and your chest. Focus on your breathing as you relax into the pose.

e. Modifications:

If it feels good to keep your knees bent in this pose, you can remain here with your calves resting. If you want to extend your legs long, you can prop them up with additional cushions. If you want to open your chest, bring your arms out to either side or bend them at a 45-degree angle. To add additional support to your lower back, you can place a pillow or bolster beneath your tailbone.

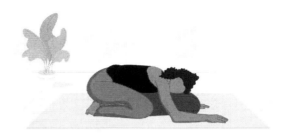

6. Child's Pose

a. Benefits:

Child's pose is a deceptively simple pose that offers a wide variety of benefits. One of these is relief from back pain. This pose elongates the spine, gently creating space between your vertebrae as you relax into the floor. After a few minutes of gentle stillness, you will start to feel your back muscles relax and soften.

b. Duration:

Hold this pose for 5 to 10 minutes.

c. Props:

- Bolster or heavy cushion

- Pillows or folded blankets

d. Instructions:

Kneel in the middle of your mat. Place a bolster or long pillow lengthwise, starting between your knees. Lower your torso down onto the prop, laying your hands out long on the mat. Ensure that your head feels supported and that your legs are comfortable. If you do not have props available, this pose is possible without them. However, you may find it difficult if you have limited mobility.

e. Modifications:

If you want to open up your shoulders in this pose, you may choose to support your forearms with blocks or cushions. For those in larger bodies or the first trimester of pregnancy, you may find it more comfortable to take a wider stance. If your hips remain raised, a wider stance may also help you access a more curved spine. Additionally, draping a heavy blanket across your hips can help to elongate the spine by pressing the hips and tailbone closer to the earth.

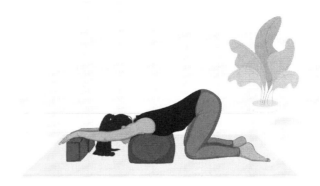

7. Melting Heart Pose

a. Benefits:

Melting heart pose is a shoulder-opening posture that addresses the upper and mid-back, while simultaneously opening the chest. This pose does a wonderful job of stretching both the back and front body. Often, shoulder and back tension is interconnected with tightness through the pectoral muscles, as our bodies rely on balance to maintain our posture throughout the day. When our mid-back muscles feel tight, there is often a chance that our chests are tight, too. Melting heart pose works on both these tight areas, providing us with the space needed to find deep, lasting relaxation.

b. Duration:

Hold this pose for 5 to 10 minutes.

c. Props:

- Yoga blocks or a stack of wide books
- Bolsters or cushions
- Pillows or folded blankets

d. Instructions:

Come to a table-top position with your hips directly above your knees and your shoulders above your hands. Make sure that your knees and your hands are a comfortable distance apart so that you do not feel crowded or constricted. Place a pillow, rolled blanket, or bolster lengthwise beneath your torso. Walk your hands forward to create more space between your knees and your palms until your hips start to come closer to the floor. Then, send your hips back until your sternum comes to rest on the props beneath you. Either rest your forehead on the floor or on a soft object such as a pillow or folded blanket. You may want to rest your upper arms on two yoga blocks for additional support. Be mindful of your shoulders and try to keep them from shrugging toward your ears. You should feel a gentle stretch through the area between your shoulder blades, as well as through your armpits, chest, and sides. Relax into the pose once you have set up your supports to your liking.

e. Modifications:

If you find that you are unable to relax fully due to your hips and glutes being unsupported, you may choose to stack pillows on your calves to act as a soft, makeshift seat. People in larger bodies may find it easier to do this pose in a wide-legged stance. As a modification, you may enjoy elevating your forearms slightly on taller blocks or bolsters. This will create more space for your chest to extend further forward. People with sensitive knees or those in the first trimester of pregnancy may find this pose easier in a standing, forward-fold position, using a counter or table to brace the arms.

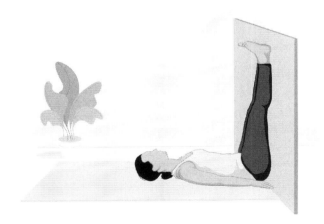

8. Legs up the Wall

a. Benefits:

This pose is one of the most addictive poses in all of restorative yoga. It looks so simple, but it packs a major relaxation punch. This pose feels incredible at the end of a busy day in particular. Legs up the wall allows your lower body to take a much-needed break from weight-bearing, using the gentle inversion to drain the legs of fluid and give your circulatory system a moment of respite. This pose offers a gentle release for your lower back and hips while using your body's own weight to massage these areas. For best results, hold this pose for more than 10 minutes to get the full benefits.

b. Duration:

Hold this pose for 10 to 20 minutes.

c. Props:

- Pillows or folded blankets
- Yoga strap or a long scarf

d. Instructions:

Place your mat or blanket near a wall or the side of a

secure piece of furniture. Take your pillow or folded blankets and place them on the ground, snug to the wall. Bring yourself close to the wall and lie on your side with your glutes pressed firmly to the wall. It may take you a moment to wiggle into position. Once you are close to the wall, swing your legs upward as you rotate onto your back and bring your hips onto the blanket or pillow. Once your legs are along the wall, vertically stacked above your hips, make sure that your lower back is supported by the props beneath you. Place a blanket across your hips and get comfortable. If you find that you are having difficulty relaxing your legs, you may find it helpful to tie them together with a yoga strap or long scarf across your thighs. This will add stability and help you fully relax.

e. Modifications:

Depending on your comfort levels, you may want to raise or lower the support beneath your low back. Add or remove supports until you find the height that feels most beneficial for your spine. Some people find it grounding to place a heavy object, such as a Magic bag or a cushion, on top of their feet. Play around with this pose to see what works best for you.

6

EXHAUSTION, BURNOUT & RESTORING ENERGY

EXHAUSTION & BURNOUT

I n today's world, we all know what exhaustion feels like. In fact, most of us actually find it harder to remember what having energy feels like because we are so used to chronic exhaustion. The demands of work, parenting, finances, education, housework, friendships, and everything else take a lot of energy. Finding a proper self-care routine that allows us to restore our energy and escape the chronic fatigue cycle can be challenging. We are constantly bombarded with conflicting information on how to tackle physical and mental exhaustion. Drink coffee! Go for a run! Take a power nap! Wading through the options can feel overwhelming when you're already feeling depleted.

When exhaustion becomes chronic, it can turn into burnout. Burnout is a term used to describe the feeling that comes when you have run out of the emotional, mental, and/or physical energy that you need to perform your basic life tasks. People in helping professions such as nurses, doctors, teachers, and social workers are more prone to developing burnout because their jobs require them to use empathy and compassion on a daily basis in the face of highly stressful challenges. Parents and overworked employees are also in danger of burning out, depending on their life and work balance. Young people, in particular, face insurmountable challenges in today's world; from balancing unpaid internships with student debt and making rent to having no clue what career path to follow, young adults also face the risk of burning out altogether when the exhausting rhythm of their lives becomes all too much. Mothers and single parents can also find themselves in this situation, feeling overworked and drained of energy because of all the different hats they have to wear each day. If your life is filled with people who rely and depend on you, with no time for your own needs or self-care, exhaustion and burnout are natural states to find yourself in.

Regardless of your circumstances, burnout sucks. It feels like even the simplest task like grocery shopping or filling out paperwork is impossible. This doesn't have to be the case, though. In the next section, I will share with you my own experiences with restorative yoga and how it helped to restore my energy.

RESTORATIVE YOGA FOR BURNOUT & EXHAUSTION

More often than not, we trick ourselves into believing that the best way to combat exhaustion or burnout is to force ourselves to down a latte, drag ourselves to the gym, or simply go to sleep to turn the world off for a brief time. While sometimes they can feel healing in an immediate sense, these strategies don't do much to address the underlying root causes of our exhaustion long-term. That is where restorative yoga comes in.

Practicing restorative yoga actually helped me to find a better sense of balance in my life as a young parent. Before, I tended to go through my days in a state of perpetual exhaustion, using brief spurts of exercise and naps as band-aids to get me through each day. Once I started restorative yoga, I was pleasantly surprised to discover that one relaxing yoga practice actually helped me to feel more energetic and less like a perpetual zombie.

Now, I manage my energy levels through restorative yoga. When I'm feeling low energy, I ask my family for an hour alone so that I can recharge. On a busy day, even thirty minutes does the trick. Rest is so vital to our well-being, especially when it comes to being present with our loved ones. In this chapter, you will learn six of my favorite poses for combating exhaustion and restoring energy.

In this section, you will learn about the following poses and their specific benefits for increasing energy and relieving exhaustion and burnout. Each pose comes with modifications to suit your needs and preferences.

1. Supported Bridge (similar variations also seen in Chapters 5 & 10)
2. Melting Heart Pose (also seen in Chapter 5)
3. Supported Fish
4. Wind-Relieving Pose (also seen in Chapters 4 & 7; also known as Knee-to-Chest Flow)
5. Supported Cobra
6. Front of the Shoulder Stretch

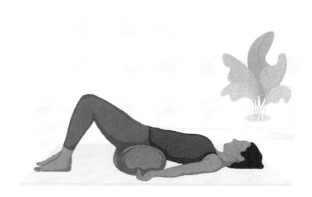

1. Supported Bridge

a. Benefits:

Supported bridge is a great pose to use when you are

feeling drained and exhausted. The gentle inversion gives your body a chance to switch gears by elevating your lower body above your head and shoulders. This subtle shift is a great way to reset your perspective and get your blood flowing throughout your body. Often when we are most tired, our minds need to see the world in a new way. This pose offers an opportunity to nourish your mind with freshly oxygenated blood while letting you take a few minutes to relax in the process. One final benefit of this pose is that the supported bridge gently applies pressure to your adrenal glands, located along your spine above your kidney region. Traditionally, it is believed that yoga poses that gently compress this area offer relief to those suffering from over-exertion.

b. Duration:

Hold this pose for 5 to 15 minutes.

c. Props:

- Pillows or cushions
- Bolster or a rolled blanket
- Yoga block or stacked books

d. Instructions:

Lie down on your back on a comfortable surface, such as a thick mat, rug, or blanket. Bend your knees and place your heels as close to your glutes as is comfortable for you. Ideally, you want your knees to be pointing toward the ceiling and for your feet to be approximately hip-width apart. Do what feels right for your body in terms of spacing. Next, slowly peel your tailbone off the floor, raising your hips to the sky one vertebra at a time. Place whatever props you have available under your hips and lower back to support your hips, ensuring that they are dense enough to keep your lower body lifted. Be mindful of your tailbone and try to keep your pubic bone tucked to create space along the lower part of your spine and across your hips. Stack your props to a height that feels comfortable and supportive. Close your eyes and relax into the pose as you breathe.

e. Modifications:

In this pose, you may find that you want more cushioning beneath your back to help you fully relax. Some people find it helpful to tie a strap or scarf around their knees so that they don't have to engage their inner thighs in this pose. If you find yourself straining in any way, consider this modification.

Depending on your comfort levels, you might opt to use a stack of books or a yoga block beneath your hips. For some people, this doesn't feel as comfortable. Notice what feels best for your body and make the necessary adjustments at the beginning to ensure the pose feels good as you sink into a relaxed state. If you are particularly drained from a lack of sleep, you may want to place a cool towel or eye mask over your face for an even deeper rejuvenating rest.

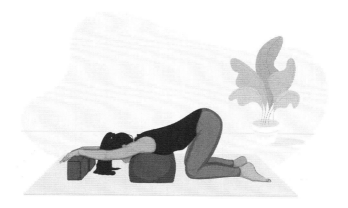

2. Melting Heart Pose

a. Benefits:

Melting heart pose is also very beneficial for combatting fatigue. Like supported bridge, this pose offers gentle compression through the adrenal glands to help stabilize the body's hormones in times of stress. From a traditional perspective, this pose focuses your energy on the heart chakra and works to open this area. When we are exhausted, this energy center can become blocked. Melting heart pose helps us to reconnect and restore our energy by opening this chakra so that our energy can flow freely. In doing so, we can access a deeper sense of gratitude and compassion, both of which help us to feel recharged and ready to step back out into the world. The physical bowing shape of the posture also lends itself to deep relaxation and helps us to completely let go of all the feelings and thoughts that weigh us down and keep us exhausted.

b. Duration:

Hold this pose for 5 to 10 minutes.

c. Props:

- Yoga blocks or a stack of wide books
- Bolsters or cushions
- Pillows or folded blankets

d. Instructions:

Come to a table-top position with your hips directly above your knees and your shoulders above your hands. Make sure that your knees and your hands are a comfortable distance apart so that you do not feel crowded or constricted. Place a pillow, rolled blanket, or bolster lengthwise beneath your torso. Walk your hands forward to create more space between your knees and your palms until your hips start to come closer to the floor. Then, send your hips back until your sternum comes to rest on the bolster or other props beneath you. Either rest your forehead on the floor or on a soft object such as a pillow or folded blanket. You may want to rest your upper arms on two yoga blocks for additional support. Be mindful of your shoulders and try to keep them from shrugging toward your ears. You should feel a gentle stretch through the area between your shoulder blades, as well as through your armpits, chest, and sides. Relax into the pose once you have set up your supports to your liking.

e. Modifications:

If you find that you are unable to relax fully due to your hips and glutes being unsupported, you may choose to stack pillows on your calves to act as a soft, makeshift seat. People in larger bodies may find it easier to do this pose in a wide-legged stance. If you have highly mobile shoulders, you may enjoy elevating your forearms slightly on taller blocks or bolsters. This modification will create more space for your chest to extend further forward. People with sensitive knees or those in the first trimester of pregnancy may find this pose easier in a standing, forward-fold position, using a counter or table to brace the arms.

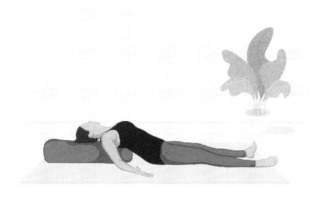

3. Supported Fish

a. Benefits:

Supported fish is a simple pose that I often crave when I'm having a tough time summoning the energy to make it through a busy week. Something about this pose just feels incredible. Fish is one part chest-opener, one part reclining relaxation. Getting into the pose is quick and easy, plus there are a variety of variations that make it extra-customizable to meet your needs on any given day. The benefits of this pose include gentle tension release through the chest, neck, and shoulders that is often caused by overwork and exhaustion. This pose in particular combats bad posture and helps you to rejoin the world in a more energetically centered and balanced state. You can use supported fish as a mid-sequence pose, or as a variation on your way to your final corpse pose at the end of your practice.

b. Duration:

Hold this pose for 5 to 20 minutes.

c. Props:

- Bolsters, couch cushions, or large pillows
- Folded blankets or rolled towels
- Weighted blanket or heavy throw
- Yoga blocks or books

d. Instructions:

Begin seated on your mat with your legs outstretched straight in front of you. Place a large pillow, bolster, or cushion behind you length-wise. Ensure that your seat is comfortable. You may want to put a folded blanket or small pillow beneath your hips if your floor is uncomfortable. Slowly lower yourself back onto the props. Allow your arms and shoulders to roll back and down until you find a comfortable release. You may choose to lay your hands on your belly or your lap as an alternative. If your head dangles off of the edge of the prop, add another pillow or cushion as support. Place a blanket across your lap and relax into the pose.

e. Modifications:

Some people like to place their legs in a butterfly position for this pose by bringing the soles of their feet to touch and letting their knees fall outward. If you choose this variation, you may want to support the outside of your knees with blocks or books.

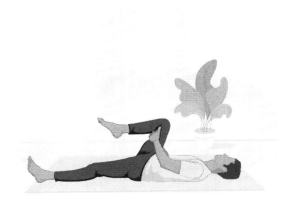

4. Wind-Relieving Pose

a. Benefits:

Wind- relieving pose has a wide variety of benefits,

including improved digestion, hip opening, and energy restoration. This pose stretches your lower back, hips, and legs while offering your internal organs a gentle, rejuvenating squeeze. This soft compression helps to wake the body and get your energetic juices flowing at times when you feel run-down or stagnant.

b. Duration:

Hold this pose for 4 to 6 minutes per side.

c. Props:

- Yoga strap or scarf
- Blanket or towel

d. Instructions:

Lie on your back. Raise one knee toward your chest. Take hold of your knee or thigh and pull your leg toward you. If your other leg begins to pop off the ground or bend, place a pillow beneath the joint. Drape a blanket or towel over your raised leg to add weight and make the pose less strenuous. Relax into the pose, gently massaging your digestive system. Repeat on both sides.

e. Modifications:

If you are pregnant or have limited mobility you may not be able to grab your leg. In this case, two variations might serve you. The first is to let your knee fall open wide to the side, rather than straight toward your torso. Hold it with one arm, rather than both. Place the other arm on the mat or rest it gently on your belly. The other variation worth trying is to take a scarf or strap and loop it around your bent leg. This will allow you to gently pull the knee toward you without any struggle. You can either hold the strap in your hands or loop it behind you to create a circle around your knee and torso.

5. Supported Cobra

a. Benefits:

This pose is the perfect antidote to feeling physically and emotionally overworked. Cobra is a very popular yoga pose across styles and it is commonly used as part of sun salutation flows. In restorative yoga, supported cobra is a variation that helps to reinvigorate the muscles along the centerline of the body while counteracting gravity's attempts to keep us hunched over and sleepy. Something about the body shape of this pose makes me feel more energetic and powerful. Plus, this pose provides a gentle core stretch as an added benefit.

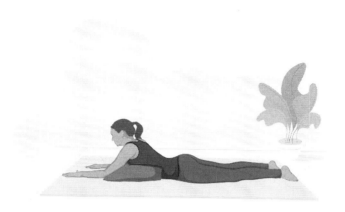

b. Duration:

Hold this pose for 5 to 10 minutes.

c. Props:

- Bolster or rolled blanket
- Small pillows or folded blankets

d. Instructions:

Lie on your stomach. Press yourself up on your forearms and slowly rise up until your chest is off the mat. Tuck your pubic bone into the mat to create space in your lower back. Slide a bolster or an alternate prop between your arms and your torso. Rest your weight on the prop and place your arms in a position on the other side that feels comfortable. Some people like to keep their arms close to 90 degrees, while others prefer to stretch them further forward. Take a deep breath and relax into the pose.

e. Modifications:

If you have a larger chest, you may find that you need a smaller prop beneath you. If you are past the first trimester of pregnancy, you may want to opt for another backbend that doesn't put pressure on your belly, such as supported fish (which is also found in this chapter).

6. Front of the Shoulder Stretch

a. Benefits:

This pose is a gentle alternative to active chest-openers. It opens the chest muscles while simultaneously allowing you to feel grounded and supported. Because this pose requires you to stay close to the ground, it allows you to regroup and restore your energy before moving on to the rest of your day. Depending on the variation, this pose also provides space for gentle core and hip stretches.

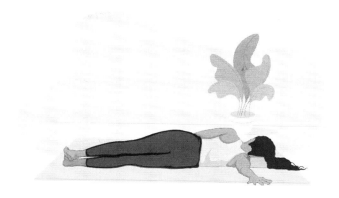

b. Duration:

Hold each side of this pose for 4 to 6 minutes.

c. Props:

- Bolster or sturdy cushions
- Pillows or folded blankets

d. Instructions:

Lie on your belly. Stretch one of your arms directly out from your shoulder, perpendicular to the long edge of the mat. Turn your palm to face the floor and press into it gently. Press your other palm into the mat beneath your shoulder and peel yourself off the mat, rolling so that your chest opens to that side of the mat. Place a bolster or pillow to support your chest in this sideways position. Rest your arm on this prop. You may choose to put another cushion or bolster beneath your top leg for stability. You should feel a stretch through your grounded arm, up through your armpit, and into your shoulder and chest. Breathe into the stretch and close your eyes to relax. Repeat on the other side.

e. Modifications:

You may find it helpful to do this pose close to the edge of a couch or next to a wall for support if your props are not sturdy enough to keep you upright throughout the duration of the pose. If you do not have ample space available, you can place your outstretched arm in a cactus position, which refers to bending your arm at a 90 degree angle.

7

INSOMNIA

Anyone who has suffered from even a mild case of insomnia knows that sleepless nights are no joke. During my postpartum period, I had a hard time falling asleep. I wasn't a chronic insomniac by any stretch, but I did experience enough sleepless nights to have a deep sense of empathy for those who struggle with the sleep disorder. In this chapter, we will explore what insomnia is, how it is caused, and how restorative yoga can help.

INSOMNIA EXPLAINED

Insomnia is a serious sleep disorder that plagues the lives of many adults and adolescents. When people suffer from insomnia they have a hard time falling asleep, often spending hours wide awake at night, frustrated and unable to rest.

Insomnia also impacts sleep quality, which means that people with insomnia wake up frequently and don't get good quality, restful sleep. Instead, they get up each morning feeling exhausted.

This sleep condition isn't just exhausting. It also comes with a whole host of side effects. People with insomnia are more likely to develop mental health issues. Many people with insomnia also have anxiety or depression. It's hard to know which comes first. Does the anxiety keep them up at night? Or does the lack of sleep cause them to feel anxious? Regardless of the cause, insomnia steals each person's ability to heal themselves properly overnight. This results in a major lack of energy and more frequent health issues. When our bodies can't rest, they can't take care of themselves properly.

Simply put, insomnia is awful. If you suffer from occasional, frequent, or chronic sleepless nights, you probably know this already. Thankfully, if we look at the most common causes of insomnia, we can see ways that restorative yoga can be used to treat this damaging disorder.

WHAT CAUSES INSOMNIA?

There isn't an easy answer when it comes to understanding why insomnia happens. Most researchers and health professionals believe that insomnia is the result of various types of stress. There are a number of ways that different forms of stress make it difficult, or even impossible, for our bodies and minds to unwind at the end of the day.

The first type of stress believed to cause insomnia is your run-of-the-mill chronic stress, be it from work, interpersonal relationships, finances, you name it. This type of stress is due to tension and problems in everyday life. Sometimes, when things get tough, our brains have a hard time letting go and switching off. If you tend to lie awake at night, scrolling through a never-ending list of responsibilities and problems, big or small, this type of stress might be the root of your insomnia.

The next form of stress that can lead to insomnia is anxiety or depression. Both of these mental health illnesses cause people to dwell on problems in their lives in fixated, troubling ways. This can cause a lot of issues when it comes to sleep because the sources of your stress can feel overwhelming and all-consuming. Trying to fall asleep while your mind swirls with worst-case scenarios can be incredibly frustrating.

Finally, the last form of stress that leads to insomnia is post-traumatic stress or post-traumatic stress disorder. When we experience trauma, our bodies go into a state of constant vigilance and arousal, meaning that we emerge from the traumatic experience unable to calm ourselves, ready for something horrible to happen at any moment. Naturally, this makes sleep difficult because our minds and bodies are constantly on edge. People who have gone through traumatic experiences often have a hard time falling asleep for this reason.

Stress comes in many forms. Regardless of the reasons you lie awake at night, your suffering is real and valid. Having been there myself, I know how hard it is to combat insomnia. I also know that healing and change are possible. Whether your insomnia is the result of a traumatic event or the stress of everyday workplace drama, restorative yoga can help you on your gentle return to a healthy sleep cycle.

RESTORATIVE YOGA FOR INSOMNIA

One of the biggest reasons people find their way to their first restorative yoga class is insomnia. It's easy to see why! The low lighting, slow movement, and focus on gentle, compassionate self-care are perfect for people who feel desperate for a little bit of rest.

There are a lot of reasons why insomniacs find restorative yoga so healing. As we have discussed already, restorative yoga teaches your body to relax and rest. For people suffering from insomnia, this is exactly what is needed to break a bad sleep cycle. Quieting a busy, overactive nervous system is the perfect antidote to stress-induced insomnia. By practicing restorative yoga, you can help your body and mind understand that you are safe, calm, and ready for rest.

In this chapter, we will look at a handful of poses that are beneficial for people suffering from insomnia. Each of these poses has a variety of benefits that will help you to relax and, ulti-mately, heal through the powers of deep, uninterrupted sleep. Each of these poses can also be done in bed, so feel free to take your insomnia-focused restorative practice to the mattress, rather than the mat. The suggested poses are listed below.

1. Sleeping Child's Pose (similar variations also seen in Chapters 5 & 9)
2. Wind-Relieving Pose (also seen in Chapters 4 & 6; also known as Knee-to-Chest Flow)
3. Supported Half Frog
4. Supported Butterfly (also seen in Chapter 8)
5. Supported Reclining Twist
6. Corpse Pose

1. Sleeping Child's Pose

a. Benefits:

This variation on a child's pose is one of my favorite moves to use when I am feeling restless at night. The upside of this variation is that it can be done directly in bed. This way, it can be used to ease yourself back into a cozy slumber when you wake up unexpectedly. Before bedtime it works as a grounding pose, letting your body know that it is time to wind down. Child's pose is one of the most comforting, secure poses in all of yoga, which makes this variation the perfect anti-dote for insomnia.

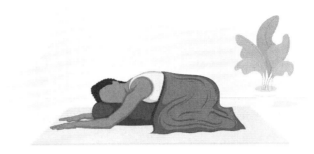

b. Duration:

Hold this pose for 5 to 10 minutes, or until you feel sleepy.

c. Props:

- Bolster or heavy cushion
- Pillows or folded blankets
- Eye mask optional
- Quilt or comforter

d. Instructions:

Come to a kneeling position in the middle of your bed. Place a bolster or long pillow lengthwise, starting between your knees. Lower your torso down onto the prop, either letting your arms fall by your sides or outstretched toward the head of your bed. Ensure that your head feels supported and that your legs are comfortable. If you do not have props available, this pose is possible without them. However, you may find it less comfortable in an unsupported pose. Pull a blanket over yourself and inhale and exhale deeply. If you have an eye mask, you may want to place it over your eyes to block out any light in your bedroom.

e. Modifications:

If you want to open up your shoulders in this pose, you may choose to support your forearms with blocks or cushions. For those in larger bodies or the first trimester of pregnancy, you may find it more comfortable to take a wider stance. If your hips remain raised, a wider stance may also help you access a more curved spine. Additionally, draping a heavy blanket across your hips can help to elongate the spine by pressing the hips and tailbone closer to the earth.

2. Wind-Relieving Pose

a. Benefits:

On top of the other benefits that wind-relieving pose has to offer, it also works wonders for treating insomnia. The compression aspect of the pose does two key things to help you get a better sleep. First, it triggers the parasympathetic nervous system by waking up your digestive tract. As you pull your knee inward, the gentle squeeze lets your brain know that it is time to settle down for the night and pay attention to your digestive tract. Second, applying pressure to your abdomen is a surefire way to help your body know that it is safe and secure. Sometimes, insomnia is caused by ongoing anxiety or the belief that we cannot rest because our attention is required. By pressing gently on your tummy, you are telling your mind that the day is over and it can let go.

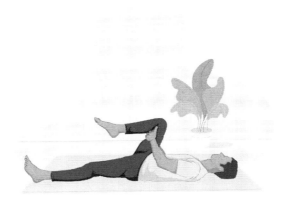

b. Duration:

Hold this pose for 4 to 6 minutes per side.

c. Props:

- Yoga strap or scarf
- Blanket or towel
- Eye mask or warm towel

d. Instructions:

Lie on your back. Raise one knee toward your chest.
Take hold of your knee or thigh and pull your leg
toward you. If your other leg begins to pop off the
ground or bend, place a pillow beneath the joint.
Drape a blanket or towel over your raised leg to add
weight and make the pose less strenuous. Relax into
the pose, gently massaging your digestive system.
Place an eye mask or a warm towel on your eyes to
block out light. Repeat on both sides.

e. Modifications:

If you are pregnant or have limited mobility you may
not be able to grab your leg. In this case, two variations might serve you. The first is to let your knee fall
open wide to the side, rather than straight toward
your torso. Hold it with one arm, rather than both.
Place the other arm on the mat or rest it gently on
your belly. The other variation worth trying is to take
a scarf or strap and loop it around your bent leg. This

will allow you to gently pull the knee toward you without any struggle. You can either hold the strap in your hands or loop it behind you to create a circle around your knee and torso.

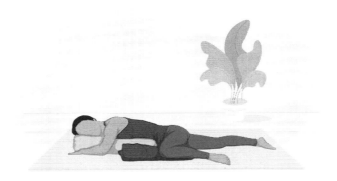

3. Supported Half Frog

a. Benefits:

This pose is grounding and calming for a variety of reasons. For people suffering from anxiety or trauma, the pressure that this pose applies to the abdomen gives a strong sense of security. Pressing the front body into the earth helps you let your body know that you are firmly rooted and safe. Our nervous systems react well to this sort of pressure, which further aids in the relaxation process. In this pose, notice the gentle press of the bolster on your heart and solar plexus chakras, as well as your root chakra. These energetic focus points will help you to feel more balanced and calm as you release into the pose.

b. Duration:

Hold this pose for 5 to 10 minutes per side.

c. Props:

- Bolster or heavy cushion
- Pillows or folded blankets
- Yoga mat or rug
- Blanket or towel

d. Instructions:

Lay a bolster or thick cushion length-wise on your mat or bed. Rest your torso, chest, and belly onto the prop. Bring one knee up to the side and turn your cheek in this direction as well. Rest your face onto the bolster and use a blanket or pillow to support your inner thigh. Place your arms in a comfortable outstretched or cactus position. Breathe deeply, feeling your belly press into the floor as you inhale. When you are finished on one side, repeat on the other for the same amount of time or breath cycles.

e. Modifications:

> If you need more cushions or support beneath your torso, adjust as needed. Play around with your arms and legs until you find a comfortable position. If you are not comfortable on your front, you can also replicate this position on your back, although it will be quite different.

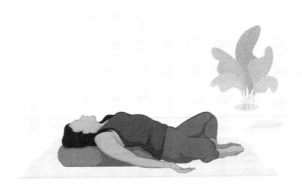

4. Supported Butterfly

a. Benefits:

> Supported butterfly is a pose that has many benefits. For starters, this pose offers instant heart-opening, both in terms of your chest muscles and your heart chakra. There is something profoundly peaceful about this pose and it always makes me feel hopeful and supported. Another benefit this pose offers is a gentle

reset to your spinal alignment. This allows for some gentle posture corrections as you rest.

b. Duration:

Hold this pose for 8 to 10 minutes.

c. Props:

- Bolster or cushion
- Pillows or folded blankets
- Blanket or towel

d. Instructions:

Sit in a butterfly position with your feet pressed together and your knees wide. Place a bolster on the ground behind you lengthwise, with one short end tucked right against your tailbone. Lower yourself backward until your back, neck, and head are rested on the bolster. Let your arms open wide, draping them on the floor. If you need support for your head, use an additional pillow or cushion. For additional grounding, drape a blanket or towel across your lap.

e. Modifications:

> To support your neck further, you can use a bolster, stack of books, or a yoga block beneath the back of your head. If your lower back feels uncomfortable, place blocks or books beneath the outside of your knees for additional support. If you are pregnant, you may find it more comfortable to be at a steeper incline. To do so, create a ramp out of additional props so that your head remains above your body, which rests back on the slope of pillows.

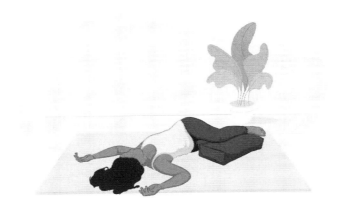

5. Supported Reclining Twist

a. Benefits:

> When you're feeling drained and restless at night, nothing beats a reclining twist. This is a powerful pose with a wide variety of awesome benefits. Some-

times, insomnia makes us feel so frustrated that it can seem almost impossible to find a comfortable position. Supported reclining twist helps your body reset and stretch out any restless jitters that might be keeping you from a restful night's sleep. Additionally, this pose draws your body's focus to your core, guiding your mind to give your digestive system some love. This helps trigger your rest and digest instincts, further aiding you in your quest for relaxation.

b. Duration:

Hold this pose for 4 to 8 minutes per side.

c. Props:

- Pillows or folded blankets
- Heavy blankets or a weighted blanket
- Bolster or cushion

d. Instructions:

Lie on your back with your arms and legs comfortably outstretched. Using your feet, gently lift your hips a few inches to the left. Raise your left leg with the knee bent at a 90-degree angle. Place a bolster alongside your right leg. Twist, lowering your left calf and thigh onto the bolster. Ensure that the prop is high enough for your leg to be supported in the twist without you needing to strain or lift your shoulder off the ground. If needed, add additional pillows or blankets. Keep your arms open at either side of your body and breathe, sinking into the twist. Feel the gentle stretch along your left hip and back as you enter into a calm, peaceful state. Repeat on the right side after 4 to 8 minutes.

e. Modifications:

If you find this stretch puts pressure on your back or if you are nervous about twisting through your spine, you can do this pose with both legs bent. Simply bend both legs to a 90-degree angle and let them fall to one side, stacking your knees on one another. If you are uncomfortable with your legs pressed together, add a pillow or folded blanket between your thighs.

6. Corpse Pose

a. Benefits:

Corpse pose is a grounding, calming pose that works wonders for restless minds. When I am worried, I find this pose very helpful as it provides comfort alongside a gentle upper body stretch. When paired with a weighted blanket or heavy quilt, corpse pose is relaxing and leaves you feeling at peace and ready for a long sleep.

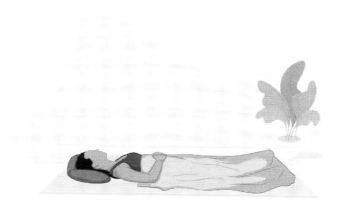

b. Duration:

Hold this pose for 1o minutes to whenever you fall asleep! Yup, it's that good.

c. Props:

- Weighted blanket or heavy quilt
- Comfortable surface such as a bed, yoga mat, or rug
- Pillows or bolsters
- Folded blanket or towel

d. Instructions:

Lie down on your back with your legs outstretched

and your head supported by a folded blanket, pillow, or towel. Bring your hands to rest on your belly or chest. If it feels comfortable, place pillows beneath your elbows to support your arms with light cushioning.

e. Modifications:

If you feel pressure on your lower back or hips, you can try a few things. One option is to place a pillow or rolled towel beneath your knees. Another option is to elevate your back slightly with a bolster or pillow. One more modification is to put a slim pillow or folded blanket beneath your lower back to create support for the natural curve of your spine.

8

DEPRESSION & ANXIETY

Depression and anxiety are horrible illnesses to deal with. Whether you are feeling jittery and on-edge all the time or feeling entirely immobilized emotionally, it is debilitating to deal with. Personally, I experienced anxiety and depression only occasionally as a kid. It wasn't until I went through childbirth that I really experienced how hopeless it can feel to deal with these issues on a day-to-day basis. I suffered from postpartum depression and anxiety for about a year after my daughter was born. I spent countless nights tossing and turning as my mind raced with a variety of fears, worst-case scenarios, and hypothetical conflicts with my kids, husband, family members—the scenarios were endless and all-consuming. I constantly felt a deep sense of paranoia that someone would break into our home and kidnap my children, causing me to dash out of my bedroom every time I heard a noise and check the locks on our doors multiple times a night. It was exhausting and felt never-ending.

My depression was just as bad. I spent many mornings lying in bed for as long as I could before my kids would basically beg me to make them breakfast. Many days felt like happiness was such a lofty and silly thing to hope for. I struggled to enjoy the things I used to, like being outside, reading books, and cooking. All I wanted to do was lie down and sleep, which is near impossible as a mother of two toddlers. These illnesses I dealt with as a new mother were completely paralyzing, leaving me feeling hopeless, guilty, and inadequate.

ANXIETY & DEPRESSION EXPLAINED

For many adults and adolescents anxiety and depression go hand-in-hand. These mental health disorders, with their constant adrenaline rushes paired with excruciating bouts of feeling entirely immobilized emotionally, can be debilitating. People who suffer from these disorders have a hard time completing simple tasks like vacuuming or washing dishes, not to mention going to work or school each day.

As you probably guessed by now, I have some good news. Restorative yoga is a fantastic way to help manage your depression and/or anxiety. In the next section, I will explain how.

HOW RESTORATIVE YOGA CAN HELP ANXIETY & DEPRESSION

One of the ways that yoga can help you effectively manage your mental health is by providing your mind with an external point of focus. During the meditation phase of your practice, you will spend your time directing your energy toward specific parts of your body, noticing every sensation that crosses your mind. This is called mindfulness and it is a powerful tool for regulating mental health. The simple act of directing our attention to something other than whatever anxious thoughts are crossing our minds is a helpful way to alleviate some of the emotional strain that these disorders cause.

Rest is a huge part of managing mental illness. Many sufferers deal with high stress levels due to both their psychological symptoms and the emotional toll of feeling unregulated. Mood swings, apathy, and agitation don't feel good. For depression, in particular, it's really helpful to spend time caring for your body and allowing it to gently rest—depression is an exhausting illness. By practicing restorative yoga, you will give your mind and body time to recuperate from all of their hard work. Simultaneously, it's important to find small ways to make yourself feel comforted and relaxed.

By practicing restorative yoga, you can give yourself time to focus on inhabiting your body in a calm, safe, restful setting.

Restorative yoga is also a gentle enough practice that it isn't intimidating for people who struggle with motivation when it comes to physical activity. When you sit down to practice restorative yoga, you know that you are capable of completing a full practice without needing to push yourself. Sometimes, the best remedy is a little bit of rest.

Below are the poses we will cover in this chapter. Each pose includes modifications, benefits, and duration for your convenience.

1. Legs up the Wall (similar variations also seen in Chapters 5, 9 & 10)
2. Supported Butterfly (also seen in Chapter 7)
3. Supported Straddle Forward Fold (also seen in Chapter 10)
4. Supine Tree
5. Supine Half Moon
6. Supported Staff
7. Supine Supported Wide-Legged Fold (similar variations also seen in Chapters 5, 9 & 10)

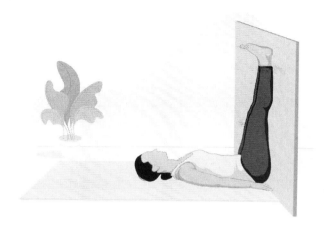

1. Legs up the Wall

a. Benefits:

One of the toughest parts of dealing with anxiety and depression can be the exhaustion that comes alongside feeling constantly low or anxious. Legs up the wall is a pose that helps to counteract feelings of heaviness and exhaustion by inverting your body and allowing your lower extremities to rest. This allows your blood to flow, your body to feel invigorated, and your emotional burden to feel less heavy.

b. Duration:

Hold this pose for 10 to 20 minutes.

c. Props:

- Pillows or folded blankets
- Yoga strap or a long scarf

d. Instructions:

Place your mat or blanket near a wall or the side of a secure piece of furniture. Take your pillow or folded blankets and place them on the ground, snug to the wall. Bring yourself close to the wall and lie on your side with your glutes pressed firmly to the wall. It may take you a moment to wiggle into position. Once you are close to the wall, swing your legs upward as you rotate onto your back and bring your hips onto the blanket or pillow. Once your legs are along the wall, vertically stacked above your hips, make sure that your lower back is supported by the props beneath you. Place a blanket across your hips and get comfortable. If you find that you are having difficulty relaxing your legs, you may find it helpful to tie them together across your thighs. This will add stability and help you fully relax.

e. Modifications:

Depending on your comfort levels, you may want to raise or lower the support beneath your low back.

Add or remove supports until you find the height that feels most beneficial for your spine. Some people find it grounding to place a heavy object, such as a Magic bag or a cushion, on top of their feet. Play around with this pose to see what works best for you.

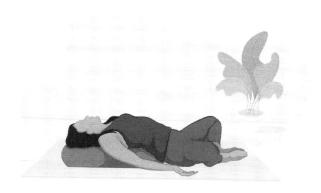

2. Supported Butterfly

a. Benefits:

An extended supported butterfly pose has many physical and emotional benefits. Physically, this pose helps you to expand through your front body, opening the chest and hips with a soft stretch. Emotionally, this pose clears pathways for energy through the heart and throat chakras. As you rest into this pose you will make way for love and gratitude to wash over you, while helping you to feel capable of communicating your feelings. For those suffering from depression and anxiety, this is a healing pose, guiding you to feel more connected and less isolated. There is strength in the pose's positioning itself, too. The vulnerability of holding your chest, arms, and hips open allows you to reach a state of acceptance and to receive new energy as you complete the pose.

b. Duration:

Hold this pose for 10 to 20 minutes.

c. Props:

- Bolster or cushion
- Pillows or folded blankets
- Blanket or towel

d. Instructions:

Sit in a butterfly position with your feet pressed together and your knees wide. Place a bolster on the ground behind you lengthwise, with one short end tucked right against your tailbone. Lower yourself backward until your back, neck, and head rest on the bolster. Let your arms open wide, draping them on the floor. If you need support for your head, use an additional pillow or cushion. For additional grounding, drape a blanket or towel across your lap.

e. Modifications:

> To support your neck further, you can use a bolster, a stack of books, or a yoga block beneath the back of your head. If your lower back feels uncomfortable, place blocks or books beneath the outside of your knees for additional support. If you are pregnant, you may find it more comfortable to be at a steeper incline. To do so, create a ramp out of additional props so that your head remains above your body, which rests back on the slope of pillows.

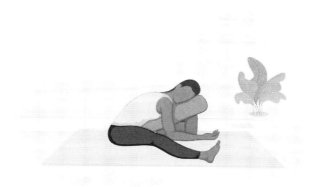

3. Supported Straddle Forward Fold

a. Benefits:

> Supported straddle forward fold is a highly beneficial pose for those combating mental health issues such as anxiety and depression. The gentle pressure on the

166 | MIA CALDWELL

abdomen, combined with the inward focus of the posture provides grounding and security. Often, people with anxiety struggle with digestion issues, so this pose is also helpful in that regard. When you are in a supported forward fold, notice your solar plexus and third eye chakras, focusing your energy on these points to increase your ability to see the world clearly and objectively and to tune in to your feelings.

b. Duration:

Hold this pose for 5 to 10 minutes.

c. Props:

- Bolsters or thick cushions (2–3)
- Blanket or towel
- Books or bolsters

d. Instructions:

Find a comfortable seat with your legs outstretched in front of you. Open your legs slightly, remaining comfortable. Stack bolsters or cushions on the floor between your legs until you can comfortably bend forward to rest your upper body on this tower of supports. Turn your face to one side to rest your cheek on your crossed arms, or, you can place your head face down, with your forehead slightly elevated by a block or pillow. Rest here, feeling a gentle stretch through your back body as well as a soft compression through your abdomen.

e. Modifications:

Depending on your body shape, flexibility, and height, this pose may look a variety of ways. If you are pregnant or in a larger body, it may be more comfortable to open your legs slightly before folding forward, so that your supports are stacked on the floor. Alternatively, this pose can be done from a seated or standing position, using a counter and a chair, if needed.

4. Supine Tree

a. Benefits:

Supine tree is a great way to ease yourself into a final corpse or savasana pose at the end of your restorative practice. This pose works to gently open your hips while allowing you to sink into the floor. Hip-opening poses are excellent to use when you are struggling with depression and anxiety as we hold a lot of emotion in our hips and sacral chakra region.

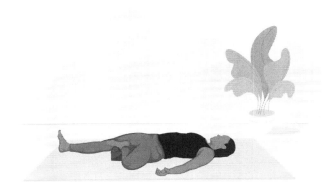

b. Duration:

Hold this pose for 5 to 10 minutes per side.

c. Props:

- Pillow or folded blanket
- Rolled towel or neck pillow
- Block or stack of books
- Blanket or towel

d. Instructions:

Bring yourself into a supine position and make your-self comfortable. Allow your legs and arms to open out to the sides in a relaxed manner. Bring your right foot onto the mat, bending at the knee as you plant your foot. Place your foot as close to your glutes or as far away as feels comfortable. Then, allow your knee to fall open to the side. Once you find a gentle stretch, place a block or books beneath the outside edge of your knee for support. Drape a blanket or towel across your hips and belly. If you want more support for your neck, place a neck pillow or rolled towel beneath your spine, supporting the natural curve of your body. Breathe deeply, releasing into the floor. Repeat on the left side when you are ready.

e. Modifications:

If you are pregnant, you may find it more comfortable to lie on an incline. In this case, stack cushions or pillows behind you before lying down. If your lower back bothers you in this pose, you can place another pillow or folded blanket beneath your outstretched leg.

5. Supine Half Moon

a. Benefits:

Supine half moon is a unique pose. Because this pose stretches your entire side body, it is a great opportunity to check in with parts of yourself that you don't always pay attention to. Similar to supine tree, this pose is wonderful for the end of a practice, before your savasana or corpse pose. As you lie on your back you may find yourself opening up and perhaps even seeing your own life in unexpected and new ways.

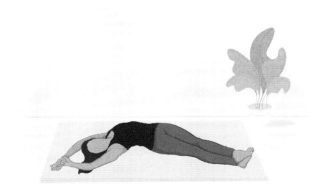

b. Duration:

Hold each side of this pose for 4 to 8 minutes.

c. Props:

- Blankets or towels
- Pillow or folded blanket

d. Instructions:

Lie down on your back. Reach your arms overhead and your legs outstretched on the mat. With your body pressed into the floor, begin to stretch your toes and your fingertips over to the right, creating the shape of a crescent moon with your body. Notice the stretch through your left ribs, hips, and arms as you reach. Find a place where you feel a stretch but can relax without needing to exert energy. Here, place a blanket over your body, keeping you snug and warm. Close your eyes and breathe, embracing the gentle stretch. Repeat on both sides.

e. Modifications:

If you feel that you need support for your lower back or neck, use a towel or pillow to provide cushioning for yourself. Additionally, if you struggle to maintain the positioning of this pose as you relax, you can place a heavy book or a weighted object in your palms or on top of your ankles to root your limbs in place. Ensure that you feel comfortable and not strained as you relax into this pose.

6. Supported Staff

a. Benefits:

This very simple pose is a wonderful way to ground yourself when you are feeling overwhelmed with negative emotions. A supported staff pose can be done anywhere there is a wall and room to sit, so you can even use this pose as a way to ground yourself if you're feeling upset or panicked in your everyday life.

Some yogis use this pose when they have panic attacks as it brings feelings of groundedness and security.

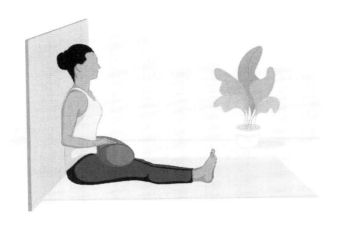

b. Duration:

Hold this pose for 5 to 10 minutes.

c. Props:

- Bolster or cushion
- Blanket or towel
- Wall to sit against

d. Instructions:

Move your mat or rug to an open wall and sit with your back pressed against the wall. Place your legs straight out in front of you. Place a bolster or heavy cushion onto your lap and rest your forearms and hands on top of it. If it helps you relax, drape a towel or blanket across your lap. Close your eyes and breathe.

e. Modifications:

If you need support for your lower back, you might find it comfortable to place a small pillow or cushion behind your tailbone and hips. Should your knees feel uncomfortable, place a folded blanket or pillow behind them. For additional grounding, you could also drape a weighted blanket across your lap if you have one available.

7. Supine Supported Wide-Legged Fold

a. Benefits:

Supine supported wide-legged fold is a great pose for those feeling drained and overwhelmed by their current circumstances. There is something very secure about this pose, perhaps due to the firm grounding of both the wall and the floor along your entire back and legs. This pose is a great one for anxiety and depression as it forces you to change your posture and open through your front body in ways that feel physically positive and optimistic. It's okay to let go of difficult emotions in this pose and completely natural to feel new and unexpected feelings bubbling to the surface as you relax and breathe. In terms of the physical benefits, this pose provides you with an inner thigh stretch as well.

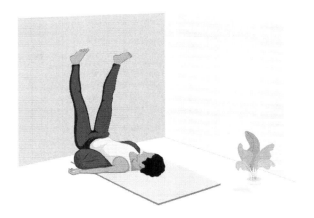

b. Duration:

Hold this pose for 10 to 15 minutes.

c. Props:

- Bolster or heavy cushion
- Blanket or towel
- Scarf, belt, or yoga strap

d. Instructions:

Find a wall and place your yoga mat with the short side along the wall. Lie down on your back in front of the wall with your legs upward, creating an L shape with your body. Your hips should be snugly pressed into the space where the floor meets the wall. Place a yoga strap or scarf around your legs at the thighs, just beneath the knees. Allow your legs to fall open until you feel a gentle stretch through your inner thighs. Then, tighten the strap so that your legs are supported and so that the stretch does not become too intense. You have the option to place a bolster or pillow beneath your hips and tailbone to support your lower back. Breathe and relax into this pose.

e. Modifications:

If you find this pose too intense, you can also tighten the strap around your legs while they are upright, preventing them from opening into a thigh stretch. If you find it hard to relax in this pose, consider wearing socks or slippers to keep your feet warm or place a heavy cushion or weighted blanket on your abdomen. If you are highly flexible, you could also place bolsters or cushions beneath the outside edges of your legs, rather than using a strap.

9

WOMEN'S POSES

RESTORATIVE YOGA FOR WOMEN

When I got pregnant with my first child, it had been a while since I had regularly practiced yoga. I had a terrible experience with my pregnancy. As much as I wanted pregnancy to be a transformative, incredible process, I felt sick, emotional, and depressed. It was so much worse than I expected it to be. I felt like I lost touch with who I was as a person as the trimesters wore on. This first pregnancy was such a difficult experience that when I got pregnant with my second child, I knew I had to do something differently.

After finding out that I was pregnant again, I decided I wanted to make my next pregnancy a better and more positive experience. Recalling the amazing experiences I had had with yoga in the past, I committed to doing prenatal yoga throughout my second pregnancy. I did it once every few weeks in the beginning but wasn't very consistent due to morning sickness and other challenges of pregnancy. Toward the end of my pregnancy, I was so uncomfortable and hardly sleeping. I started doing yoga almost every night before I went to sleep and it was the only thing that helped me fall asleep totally relaxed.

Months later, as a new mom of two, I began to experience a deep postpartum depression that really threw me. I felt completely unhappy and could hardly get myself out of bed. Realizing that I had to find a way out of the rut I was in, I sought help from my doctor and I turned back to yoga. I don't even know what it was, but something within me "awoke," as if it clicked then and there that yoga would be the thing that would save me from myself. I began practicing yoga multiple times each week and committed to doing restorative yoga once a week to allow myself to rest.

When I find myself in the throes of menstrual cramps or overwhelmed by the demands of motherhood, yoga is always there for me. As a woman and a mother, I have learned first-hand that yoga is a powerful tool for self-preservation and self-care. As women, we give so much of ourselves to the people and the causes we are passionate about that we some-times forget to take time for ourselves.

When I set out to write this book, one of the first things that I struggled with was how to explain all the ways that I have found restorative yoga healing as a woman. In this section, I will share the ways it can help in three distinctly challenging parts of the female experience: pregnancy, menstruation, and menopause.

RESTORATIVE YOGA FOR PREGNANCY

Growing a human is an incredible, unique, sometimes baffling experience. Morning sickness, body aches, and exhaustion take their toll on expectant mothers, leaving us drained and weary. It can be really hard to adjust to all of the changes in your body throughout pregnancy, too. For many women, exercise is also a challenge, especially if you are experiencing a high-risk pregnancy.

Restorative prenatal yoga is a fabulous way to care for your body as it does the awe-inspiring job of nurturing your baby. By including prenatal restorative practice into your daily routine throughout your pregnancy, you can ease your aches and pains while keeping your stress levels as low as possible. Because restorative yoga is such a gentle practice, it is generally considered a safe way for pregnant women to find relief. Be sure to check in with your doctor before beginning a restorative yoga practice during your pregnancy. Listen to your body and make any changes needed to ensure that these poses feel safe and comfortable.

The following poses listed are the ones we will explore for pregnancy. Each pose has instructions, modifications, and benefits.

1. Legs up the Wall (First Trimester Only; similar variation also seen in Chapters 5, 8, 9 & 10)
2. Wide-Legged Forward Fold with Chair
3. Supported Malasana
4. Supported Seated Butterfly

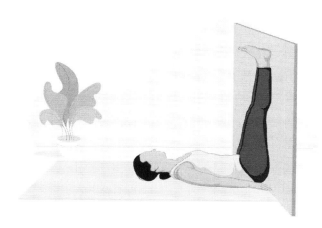

1. Legs up the Wall (First Trimester Only)

a. Benefits:

During pregnancy, many women find that their legs and feet begin to swell. This, paired with carrying extra weight around, is challenging for your body and can feel pretty terrible. This pose allows you to take a break and helps your body to release some of the fluid trapped in your lower extremities. On a less technical note, it also just feels really good to put your feet up for a while.

b. Duration:

Hold this pose for 10 to 20 minutes.

c. Props:

- Pillows or folded blankets
- Yoga strap or a long scarf

d. Instructions:

Place your mat or blanket near a wall or the side of a secure piece of furniture. Take your pillow or folded blankets and place them on the ground, snug to the wall. Bring yourself close to the wall and lie on your side with your glutes pressed firmly to the wall. It may take you a moment to wiggle into position. Once you are close to the wall, swing your legs upward as you rotate onto your back and bring your hips onto the blanket or pillow. Once your legs are along the wall, vertically stacked above your hips, make sure that your lower back is supported by the props beneath you. Place a blanket across your hips and get comfortable. If you find that you are having difficulty relaxing your legs, you may find it helpful to tie them together across your thighs. This will add stability and help you fully relax.

e. Modifications:

Depending on your comfort levels, you may want to raise or lower the support beneath your low back. Add or remove supports until you find the height that feels most beneficial for your spine. Some people find it grounding to place a heavy object, such as a Magic bag or a cushion, on top of their feet. If you are experiencing morning sickness, you may want to place a cool cloth on your brow. Play around with this pose to see what works best for you.

2. Wide-Legged Forward Fold with Chair

a. Benefits:

This forward fold is a wonderful pregnancy-safe variation. This pose takes pressure off of your lower back, which many women find to be painful during pregnancy. In addition, it allows you to gently stretch your leg muscles and hips, which often become quite sore.

b. Duration:

Hold this pose for 4 to 8 minutes.

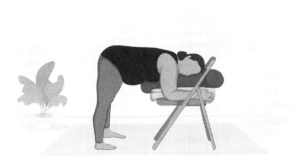

c. Props:

- Chair without wheels
- Bolster or heavy cushion
- Folded blankets or pillows

d. Instructions:

Stand in front of a chair with your feet more than shoulder-width apart. Place bolsters and pillows onto the chair, creating a sturdy cushioning to a height that feels right for your body. Fold forward, lowering your head and arms onto these supports. Adjust your props until you feel secure and able to release any tension in your back. Breathe, resting into the pose as you stretch through the backs of your legs.

e. Modifications:

Bring your feet closer together or further apart depending on your flexibility level. This pose is accessible for any body size.

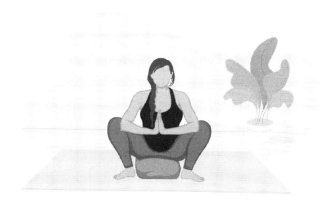

3. Supported Malasana

a. Benefits:

Supported Malasana is a fantastic pose for expecting women. This amazing hip-opener gets you in touch with your feminine side while helping your body prepare for the changes to come as you move toward labor. The shape of this pose replicates the squatting position that women have taken during childbirth since the beginning of time. It is grounding, releases lower back pressure, and reminds you that your body

184 | MIA CALDWELL

is strong, wise, and capable. During this pose, focus on your sacral and root chakras.

b. Duration:

Hold this pose for 5 to 10 minutes, depending on your comfort levels.

c. Props:

- Blocks or books
- Pillows or folded blankets

d. Instructions:

Stand with your feet hip-width apart, or a little wider. Turn your feet out to the sides so that they point to the corners of your mat. Ensure that your knees follow, turning out in line with your feet and hips. Beneath you, place a block or multiple blocks to a height that you will feel comfortable squatting to. You may want to top the block(s) with a blanket or pillow to make the surface soft and comfortable to sit on. Lower your hips onto the block, assuming a deep squat position. Press your elbows into your thighs, bringing your hands into a prayer position. Breathe in and out, feeling your thighs and hips open as you sink lower, feeling peaceful and powerful.

e. Modifications:

If you are in the second or third trimester, you may feel a bit off-balance in this pose due to your growing belly. If this is the case, you may want to do this pose with your back pressed against a wall or large piece of furniture for support. This is a nice way to ensure that you feel secure and stable as you relax into the pose.

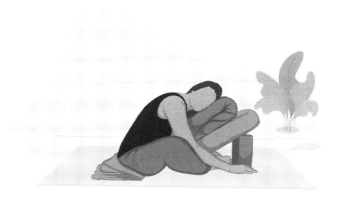

4. Supported Seated Butterfly

a. Benefits:

This pose offers a gentle stretch for your hips and glutes. During pregnancy, your muscles are working overtime to keep your changing body upright and stable. This pose gives them a brief break and offers some soft love and care to your lower body while keeping your baby safe from any unnecessary compression through your torso.

b. Duration:

Hold this pose for 10 to 20 minutes.

c. Props:

- Bolsters or heavy cushions
- Blankets or towels
- Optional: a coffee table or lap table

d. Instructions:

Sit on your mat in a comfortable position with your legs outstretched. Bring the soles of your feet to touch, allowing your legs to fall into a butterfly position. Create support for your upper body with cushions or bolsters and bring your chest and head to rest on these supports. Lean into the supports, stretching softly through your thighs and hips. If you turn your head to one side, make sure to switch your gaze halfway through the pose. Breathe.

e. Modifications:

If you need a lot of space for your belly, sit in front of

a coffee table or a lap table to create that extra room. Place soft supports on top of this surface. This modification will allow you to continue this pose into your second and third trimesters. If you feel uncomfortable sitting on a mat for this long, use a cushion or pillow beneath you.

RESTORATIVE YOGA FOR MENSTRUAL CRAMPING

Cramps are horrible. There is no denying it. You're having a great day and then suddenly, your entire abdomen is leading a mutiny against the rest of your body. In this section, we will go over poses that will help you get through your period pain-free. Each pose offers specific relief from cramping and can be done with a hot water bottle, Magic bag, or heated blanket. Be gentle with yourself and adjust the poses until they feel right for your body. The poses listed below are the ones we will cover in this section.

1. Legs up the Wall (similar variations also seen in Chapters 5, 8 & 10)
2. Wide-Legged Child's Pose (similar variations also seen in Chapters 5 & 7)
3. Supported Open Twist
4. Supported Seated Butterfly

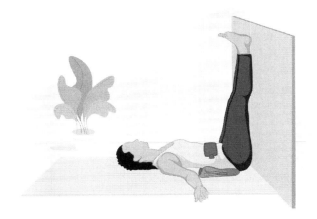

1. Legs up the Wall

a. Benefits:

Legs up the wall is a fantastic pose when it comes to dealing with menstrual cramps. The combination of a gentle inversion with lower back and hip massage works wonders for taking your mind off of your cramps. I find that this pose is especially helpful during the first few days of my period, as it is gentle and effective.

b. Duration:

Hold this pose for 10 to 20 minutes.

c. Props:

- Pillows or folded blankets

- Yoga strap or a long scarf
- Magic bag, heating pad, or hot water bottle

d. Instructions:

Place your mat or blanket near a wall or the side of a secure piece of furniture. Take your pillow or folded blankets and place them on the ground, snug to the wall. Bring yourself close to the wall and lie on your side with your glutes pressed firmly to the wall. It may take you a moment to wiggle into position. Once you are close to the wall, swing your legs upward as you rotate onto your back and bring your hips onto the blanket or pillow. Once your legs are along the wall, vertically stacked above your hips, make sure that your lower back is supported by the props beneath you. Place a blanket across your hips and get comfortable. If you find that you are having difficulty relaxing your legs, you may find it helpful to tie them together across your thighs. This will add stability and help you fully relax. Finally, if you have a Magic bag, heating pad, or hot water bottle, place it upon your abdomen or, if you prefer, beneath your lower back. Let yourself relax into the pose and enjoy a few minutes cramp-free.

e. Modifications:

> Depending on your comfort levels, you may want to
> raise or lower the support beneath your low back.
> Add or remove supports until you find the height that
> feels most beneficial for your spine. If your cramps
> are particularly bad, you may find it preferable to
> keep your Magic bag or hot water bottle under your
> back, rather than on top of your abdomen. Some
> people find it grounding to place a heavy object, such
> as a Magic bag or a cushion, on top of their feet. Play
> around with this pose to see what works best for you.

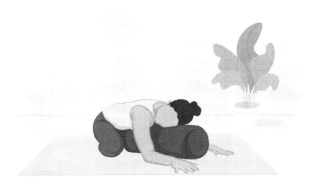

2. Wide-Legged Child's Pose

a. Benefits:

> One of the most amazing benefits of child's pose is the
> relief it provides from menstrual cramps. Doing this

pose in a wide-legged position allows more space for your abdomen as well as a gentle hip, back, and leg stretch. These combined sensations work wonders for taking your mind off of nagging aches.

b. Duration:

Hold this pose for 5 to 15 minutes

c. Props:

- Bolster or heavy cushion
- Pillows or folded blankets
- Hot water bottle, electric blanket, or Magic bag

d. Instructions:

Come to a kneeling position in the middle of your mat. Place a bolster or long pillow lengthwise, starting between your knees. Lower your torso down onto the prop, laying your hands out long on the mat. Ensure that your head feels supported and that your legs are comfortable. If you do not have props available, this pose is possible without them. However, you may find it difficult if you have limited mobility.

e. Modifications:

> For added pain relief, use a Magic bag, electric blanket, or hot water bottle on top of your bolster or pillow. Ensure that your abdomen comes to rest on it as you lower down. Alternatively, you may want to place this warm object on your lower back once you are in the pose.

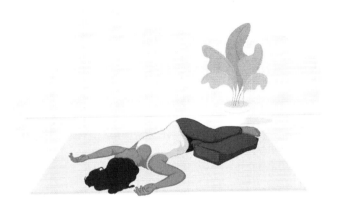

3. Supported Open Twist

a. Benefits:

> The benefits of supported open twist include relief from lower back pain due to cramping, as well as gentle stretching across your abdomen, which is working hard as you move through your monthly cycle. The twisting motion of this pose also helps to

alleviate pressure on your lower back while redirecting your body's attention elsewhere.

b. Duration:

Hold this pose for 5 to 10 minutes per side.

c. Props:

- Magic bag or hot water bottle
- Bolster or cushion
- Pillows or folded blankets

d. Instructions:

Lie down on your back with your feet planted and your knees bent. Drop your knees to one side, twisting through your mid-back. Place a bolster or a cushion between your legs to offer some stability and support. Put a warm prop such as a Magic bag, electric blanket, or hot water bottle either behind your low back or on top of your lower abdomen, depending on the placement that feels most beneficial to you. Breathe here, exhaling to release tension through your belly. If you wish, place a blanket over yourself, or a pillow beneath your head. After 5 to 10 minutes, switch slowly to the other side, mindfully transitioning without any sudden movements that might increase your cramping.

e. Modifications:

Make any small adjustments needed to alleviate cramping. If you find that you are slightly nauseous due to the intensity of your symptoms, you can incline your body slightly on a bolster or large couch cushion.

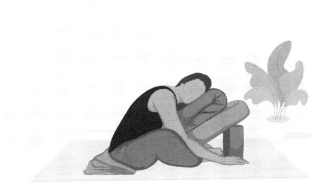

4. Supported Seated Butterfly

a. Benefits:

This pose offers a gentle stretch for your hips and glutes. During menstrual cramps, your muscles are working overtime to support your reproductive cycle. This pose

gives those muscles a brief break and offers some soft
love and care to your lower body. This pose is best for
minor cramping, rather than intense cramps, as it does
include some slight compression of the abdomen, so use
your discretion when including this pose in a flow.

b. Duration:

Hold this pose for 10 to 20 minutes.

c. Props:

- Bolsters or heavy cushions
- Blankets or towels
- Magic bag, hot water bottle, or heated blanket

d. Instructions:

Sit on your mat in a comfortable position with your
legs outstretched. Bring the soles of your feet to
touch, allowing your legs to fall into a butterfly position. Create support for your upper body with cushions or bolsters and bring your chest and head to rest
on these supports. Lean into the supports, stretching
softly through your thighs and hips. If you turn your
head to one side, make sure to switch your gaze
halfway through the pose. If you want some addi-

tional relief, use a heated prop on your abdomen. Breathe.

e. Modifications:

As with the previous poses, make any adjustments you feel are helpful for your body in its current state. Some women find it helpful to sit on a cushion or meditation pillow to elevate their hips.

RESTORATIVE YOGA FOR MENOPAUSE

Menopause is a challenging phase in a woman's life. Hot flashes, heightened anxiety, mood swings, and insomnia are just a few of the obstacles this transitional time brings up for most women. Restorative yoga can help you manage your menopause symptoms as you make your way through this emotional and physical rollercoaster ride.

The poses listed below are the ones that we will cover for menopause. Each of these poses will include the benefits and instructions on how to do them.

1. Supported Locust
2. Supported Pigeon
3. Reclining Half Hero
4. Heart Pose with Butterfly Legs (also seen in Chapters 7, 8 & 10)

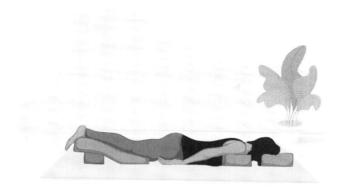

1. Supported Locust

a. Benefits:

Supported locust is a wonderful pose for when you
need a major refresh. This pose stretches the front
body, which is great for when you're feeling frustrated, stressed, or overheated. By slightly elevating
the upper and lower body, this pose helps you to reset
your posture and open through the chest and hips.

b. Duration:

Hold this pose for 5 to 10 minutes.

c. Props:

- Bolsters or cushions
- Blocks or books

- Folded blankets or pillows
- Cold compress or cool cloth

d. Instructions:

Come to your mat and lie on your belly. Place a bolster or cushion beneath your upper chest and shoulders to slightly elevate your upper body. Place either a block or books beneath your forehead to support your head and neck. Under your shins, place another bolster to elevate your legs, stretching your hip flexors and quads gently. If you are feeling heated, you can opt to place a cold compress on the back of your neck for additional relief. Breathe deeply and sink into the floor. Let your arms find a natural location that feels comfortable.

e. Modifications:

If the incline is too intense, use folded blankets or pillows in place of bolsters.

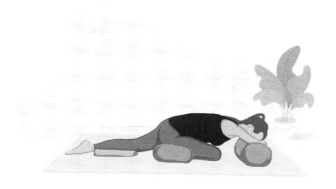

2. Supported Pigeon

a. Benefits:

Restorative versions of pigeon pose are a fantastic way to open the hips and restore flexibility to your body when you are feeling stiff and overwhelmed. This pose opens your legs and hips to help you feel limber and mobile day to day.

b. Duration:

Hold each side of this pose for 5 to 10 minutes.

c. Props:

- Bolsters or cushions
- Cool cloth or compress
- Pillow or folded blanket

d. Instructions:

Bring yourself into a table-top position on all fours on your mat. Place a bolster in front of your knees and a pillow beneath your left shin. Put another bolster in front of your hands so that you can grab it when needed. Lift your right leg, bringing your right knee behind your right wrist. Lay your right calf down on the floor in front of the bolster, resting your right thigh on the bolster. Lower your upper body down onto the second bolster until you find a comfortable position. Relax into the pose, feeling a stretch through your outer hips, glutes, and thighs. Repeat on the opposite side. Use a cool cloth or compress on the back of your neck if you feel warm.

e. Modifications:

Adjust your shin to find a position that feels comfortable for the duration of the pose. If you feel like this pose is a bit too intense, place more than one bolster under your front thigh for additional support.

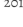

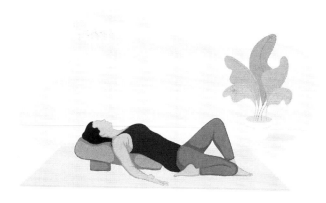

3. Reclining Half Hero

a. Benefits:

This pose has a variety of benefits, from energy restoration to front body opening. In reclining half hero pose, you will feel your worries and tension melt away as you sink into the floor. For women struggling with menopause symptoms, this pose helps you feel rejuvenated and refreshed when things feel out of control. While relaxing into this gentle stretch, pay attention to your heart chakra, which is a focal point for this pose.

b. Duration:

Hold each side of this pose for 5 to 10 minutes.

c. Props:

- Bolster or cushion
- Blocks or books
- Pillows or folded blankets

d. Instructions:

Place a yoga block on your mat, with a bolster on it to create an inclined slope. Kneel in front of these props, placing a folded blanket underneath your right shin. Straighten your left leg and place your foot on the floor to brace as you lower backward onto the props you've prepared. Ensure that your neck feels supported and that the incline is high enough for you to feel stable and secure. Breathe deeply and relax before transitioning to the other side.

e. Modifications:

If you feel like this pose is intense on your knee joint, you can place a folded blanket behind your knee to create space between your thigh and calf. Alternatively, you can also lean against a wall rather than piling props, if you feel like you need more stability and want to be upright.

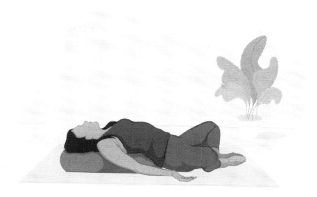

4. Supported Butterfly

a. Benefits:

Supported butterfly is a gentle chest-opener and backbend that will help you regulate your breathing and body temperature during adrenaline rushes and hot flashes. This heart pose variation is calming as it allows you to fully sink back into the pose while expanding your front body, making space for deep, soothing, expansive breaths.

b. Duration:

Hold this pose for 5 to 15 minutes.

c. Props:

- Bolster or firm cushion

- Blocks, sturdy pillows, or books
- Blanket or towel

d. Instructions:

Sit on your mat with your legs in a butterfly position with your feet pressed to one another and your knees wide. Place a bolster or firm cushion about two hands' lengths away from your glutes. Put blocks, pillows, or books beneath the outside of your knees to support your legs. Slowly roll back onto the mat, bringing your back to rest on the bolster. Make sure that the bolster begins beneath your shoulder blades and continues upward to support your head. Breathe deeply and allow your arms to fall to the sides.

e. Modifications:

You may find it grounding and comforting to place your hands on your abdomen if you feel particularly jittery or stressed. Additionally, a blanket draped across your lap can create a similar calming effect.

10

STRESS RELIEF

By this point in the book, I'm sure you feel like an expert in restorative yoga and why it works so well to manage stress. For this chapter, I've kept the introduction brief because you already know the basics. Stress is terrible and plagues so many of our lives because of how we live in today's modern world. Family responsibilities, challenging financial situations, and long hours mean that many of us feel overworked and overwhelmed by all the hats we have to wear each day. Left unmanaged, stress can lead to a variety of physical and mental health problems.

As you may have guessed, restorative yoga works wonders when it comes to managing and mitigating stress. The calming breathwork, paired with the long, relaxing poses, combine to create the perfect antidote to a stressed-out mind. In this section, I will show you poses that can help you manage your stress effectively.

Here are the poses we will discuss in this chapter:

1. Heart Pose with Butterfly Legs (also seen in Chapter 9)
2. Supported Straddle Forward Fold (also seen in Chapter 8)
3. Extended Supported Bridge (similar variations also seen in Chapters 5 & 6)
4. Supported Backbend with Legs up the Wall (similar variations also seen in Chapters 5, 8 & 9)
5. Reclining Butterfly with Supported Feet
6. Restorative Frog

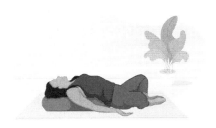

1. Supported Butterfly

a. Benefits:

Supported butterfly is a gentle chest-opener and

backbend. When we are stressed out, we tend to hunch forward and constrict our breathing. This creates a self-perpetuating cycle of stress as our body becomes habituated to shallow, restricted breathing. Not to mention the fact that hunching over feels terrible long-term. This heart pose variation is calming as it allows you to fully sink back into the pose while expanding your front body, making space for deep, soothing, expansive breaths.

b. Duration:

Hold this pose for 5 to 15 minutes.

c. Props:

- Bolster or firm cushion
- Blocks, sturdy pillows, or books
- Blanket or towel

d. Instructions:

Sit on your mat with your legs in a butterfly position with your feet pressed to one another and your knees wide. Place a bolster or firm cushion about two hands' lengths away from your glutes. Put blocks, pillows, or books beneath the outside of your knees to support your legs. Slowly roll back onto the mat, bringing your back to rest on the bolster. Make sure that the bolster begins beneath your shoulder blades and continues upward to support your head. Breathe deeply and allow your arms to fall to the sides.

e. Modifications:

You may find it grounding and comforting to place your hands on your abdomen if you feel particularly jittery or stressed. Additionally, a blanket draped across your lap can create a similar calming effect.

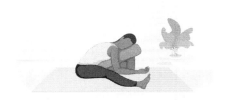

2. Supported Straddle Forward Fold

a. Benefits:

Supported straddle forward fold is a highly beneficial pose for those combating acute stress. The gentle pressure on the abdomen, combined with the inward focus of the posture provides grounding and security.

Often, people under a lot of stress deal with digestion issues, so this pose is also helpful in that regard. When you are in a supported forward fold, notice your solar plexus and third eye chakras, focusing your energy on these points to increase your ability to see the world clearly and objectively and to tune in to your feelings.

b. Duration:

Hold this pose for 5 to 10 minutes.

c. Props:

- Bolsters or thick cushions (2–3)
- Blanket or towel
- Books or bolsters

d. Instructions:

Find a comfortable seat with your legs outstretched in front of you. Open your legs slightly, remaining comfortable. Stack bolsters or cushions on the floor between your legs until you can comfortably bend forward to rest your upper body on this tower of supports. Turn your face to one side to rest your cheek on your crossed arms, or, you can place your head face down, with your forehead slightly elevated by a block or pillow. Rest here, feeling a gentle stretch through your back body as well as a soft compression through your abdomen.

e. Modifications:

Depending on your body shape, flexibility, and height, this pose may look a variety of ways. If you are pregnant or in a larger body, it may be more comfortable to let your legs open slightly before folding forward, so that your supports are stacked on the floor. Alternatively, this pose can be done from a seated or standing position, using a counter and a chair, if needed.

3. Extended Supported Bridge

a. Benefits:

Extended supported bridge is a great pose to use when you are feeling stressed out. The gentle inversion gives your body a chance to switch gears by elevating your lower body above your head and shoulders. This subtle shift is a great way to reset your perspective and get your blood flowing throughout your body. Often when we are overwhelmed, our minds need to see the world in a new way. This pose offers an opportunity to nourish your mind with freshly oxygenated blood while letting you take a few minutes to relax in the process. One final benefit of this pose is that the supported bridge gently applies pressure to your adrenal glands, located along your spine above your kidney region. Traditionally, it is believed that yoga poses that gently compress this area offer relief to those suffering from over-exertion and chronic stress.

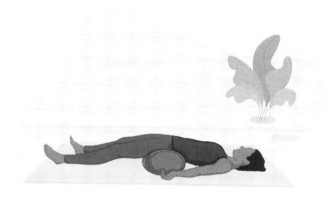

b. Duration:

Hold this pose for 5 to 15 minutes.

c. Props:

- Pillows or cushions
- Bolster or rolled blanket
- Yoga block or stacked books

212 | MIA CALDWELL

d. Instructions:

Lie down on your back on a comfortable surface, such as a thick mat, rug, or blanket. Bend your knees and place your heels as close to your glutes as is comfortable for you. Ideally, you want your knees to be pointing upward toward the ceiling and for your feet to be approximately hip-width apart. Do what feels right for your body in terms of spacing. Next, slowly peel your tailbone off the floor, raising your hips to the sky one vertebra at a time. Place whatever props you have available under your hips and lower back to support your hips, ensuring that they are dense enough to keep your lower body lifted. Be mindful of your tailbone and try to keep your pubic bone tucked to create space along the lower part of your spine and across your hips. Stack your props to a height that feels comfortable and supportive. Finally, extend your legs to lengthen the bridge and increase the stretch. Your body should be long, but the pressure should not be intense on your lower back. Close your eyes and relax into the pose as you breathe.

e. Modifications:

In this pose, you may find that you want more cushioning beneath your back to help you fully relax.

Some people find it helpful to tie a strap or scarf around their knees so that they don't have to engage their inner thighs in this pose. If you find yourself straining in any way, consider this modification. Depending on your comfort levels, you might opt to use a stack of books or a yoga block beneath your hips. For some people, this doesn't feel as comfortable. Notice what feels best for your body and make the necessary adjustments at the beginning to ensure the pose feels good as you sink into a relaxed state.

4. Supported Backbend with Legs up the Wall

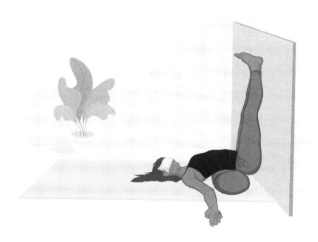

a. Benefits:

This variation on legs up the wall is an awesome way to end a stressful day. The benefits of this pose are numerous. Opening through your chest helps you to release your worries and the tension that accumulates across your shoulders during stressful times. The elevation of your legs is great for your nervous system, helping your body drain fluid from your tired lower extremities.

b. Duration:

Hold this pose for 10 to 20 minutes to fully enjoy all of the benefits.

c. Props:

- Bolster or cushion
- Eye pillow or face cloth
- Yoga strap or scarf

d. Instructions:

Move your mat to a wall. Place a bolster beneath your mid-back as you lower onto the floor and swing your legs up along the wall. Scooch close to the wall so that your hips are snug to the space where the wall meets the floor. Drape a cloth or eye pillow over your eyes and relax into the pose.

e. Modifications:

If you find it hard to keep both your legs upright, you can place a yoga strap or scarf around your legs to tie them together.

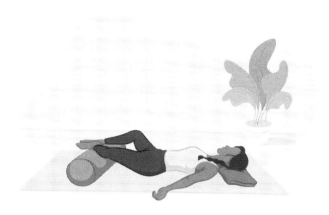

5. Reclining Butterfly with Supported Feet

a. Benefits:

This extended, slightly modified supported butterfly pose has many physical and emotional benefits. Physically, this pose helps you to expand through your front body, opening the chest and hips with a soft stretch. Emotionally, this pose clears pathways for energy through the heart and throat chakras. In this variation, the raised positioning of your feet will offer a gentle inversion and release stress through your lower extremities. Inversions are a wonderful way to change your body's current state by giving your tired feet and heart a rest.

b. Duration:

Hold this pose for 10 to 20 minutes.

c. Props:

- Bolster or cushion
- Pillows or folded blankets
- Blanket or towel

d. Instructions:

Sit in a butterfly position with your feet pressed together and your knees wide. Place a bolster underneath your feet and ankles, so that your legs are inclined slightly upward from your hips to your toes. Lie back, placing a pillow or folded blanket under your head. Let your arms open wide, draping them on the floor. For additional grounding, drape a blanket or towel across your lap. Breathe and let go of your stress as you sink into the pose.

e. Modifications:

To support your neck further, you can use a bolster, stack of books, or yoga block beneath the back of your head. If your lower back feels uncomfortable, place blocks or books beneath the outside of your knees for additional support. If you are pregnant, you may find it more comfortable to be at a steeper incline. To do so, create a ramp out of additional props so that your head remains above your body, which rests back on the slope of pillows.

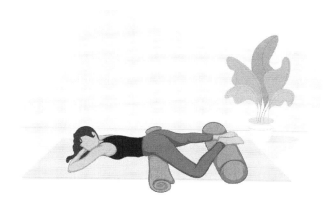

6. Restorative Frog

a. Benefits:

Restorative frog is a unique, highly beneficial pose that challenges both your mind and body. Think of this pose like a reverse supine butterfly. As you ease into the pose slowly, feel yourself grounding and opening into the earth. This pose allows you to feel simultaneously secure and challenged with a gentle, hip-opening stretch.

b. Duration:

Hold this pose for 5 to 10 minutes.

c. Props:

- Rolled blanket or towel
- Bolster or cushion

d. Instructions:

Roll a towel or blanket and place it horizontally across your mat. About one foot past this prop, place a bolster running parallel. Lower your hips onto the rolled blanket or towel, opening your knees, and rest your feet on the bolster. Adjust the props until you feel comfortable. Breathe and release into the floor. If you feel you need a pillow or a blanket to rest your head on, you can grab one as well.

e. Modifications:

Feel free to use a lower pillow or folded blanket in

place of a bolster if your feet don't feel good at such a high elevation. If your elbows don't feel comfortable, you can place a blanket or pillow beneath your upper body as well.

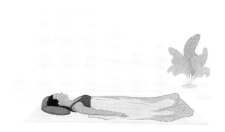

7. Savasana

a. Savasana is a pose used at the end of most yoga sequences. It is highly beneficial in reducing stress as it is known to calm the mind as well as your central nervous system. It is normal to drift away during this pose, or even fall asleep, due to its calming nature. This is also a great position to practice body scan meditation.

b. Duration:

Hold this pose for 5 to 10 minutes, or as long as you want.

c. Props:

- Blanket
- Folded blanket or soft pillow
- Bolster or cushion

d. Instructions:

Place a folded blanket or soft pillow at the top of your mat to rest your head on. Slowly lie down onto the mat, gently relaxing your head onto the padding. Bend your knees slightly and place a bolster or cushion underneath your legs. If desired, drape a blanket over your body for added comfort. Allow your arms to lie by your side. Close your eyes, and begin to breathe into the pose. Let your body fully relax here, letting go of any stress or tension you may feel.

e. Modifications:

If you feel any tension or pain in your lower back you can place a small folded blanket or cushion underneath your tailbone. Move it around until you are getting the support you need. You can keep your arms down at your side, or if you wish to create a deeper stretch in your chest, bring them out perpendicular to your body, creating a T shape. You can also try bending your arms into a cactus position, which is a 90-degree angle with your hands pointing upward. Play around with what feels good for your body. If you are pregnant, this position is best in your first trimester only. If you are in the second or third trimester, you can elevate your back by stacking props underneath you.

SEQUENCES

This section includes sequences for a variety of purposes. Some are long and some art short, designed to cater to your specific needs. You will see the images of each pose back to back and then a written order of each sequence. For a more thorough explanation of each individual meditation, pranayama, or pose, refer to earlier sections of the book where they are described in detail. The durations provided are rough estimates. Take as much or as little time as you need for your practice to feel complete.

BEGINNER'S HOLISTIC RESTORATIVE SEQUENCE

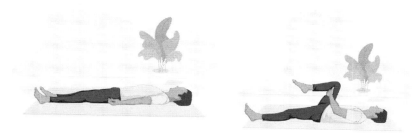

Knee-to-Chest Flow

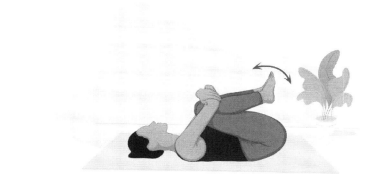

Low Back Massage Flow

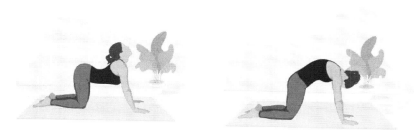

Cat and Cow Flow

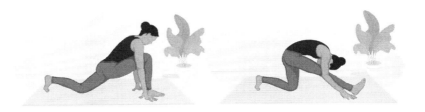

Low Lunge to Forward Fold Flow

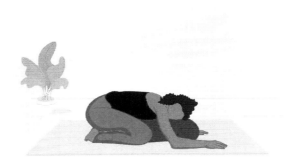

Child's Pose

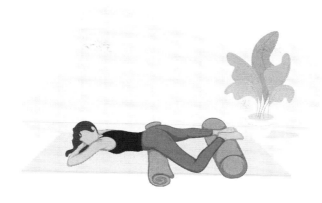

Restorative Frog

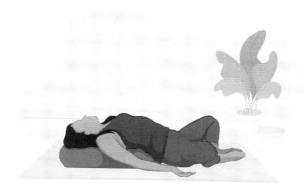

Supported Butterfly

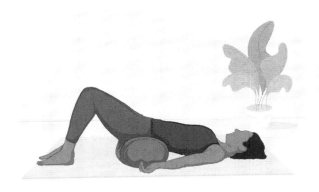

Supported Bridge

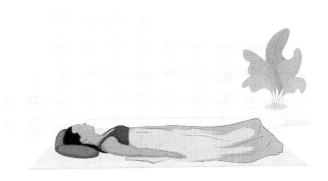

Savasana

a. Purpose:

This sequence is designed as an introductory sequence for new restorative yogis. Use this sequence to guide yourself through a holistic basic practice that covers all the bases, including stress relief, relaxation, energy restoration, and grounding. This practice can be done at any time of the day.

b. Duration:

60 minutes

c. Sequence:

- Pranayama: Balanced Breath (~5 minutes): *See Chapter 3*
- Meditation: Body Scan (~5 minutes) *See Chapter 3*
- Warm-Up: (~10 minutes) *See Chapter 4*
- Knee-to-Chest Flow
- Low Back Massage Flow
- Cat and Cow Flow
- Low Lunge to Forward Fold Flow
- Child's Pose (~5 minutes) *See Chapters 5, 7 & 9*
- Restorative Frog (~5 minutes) *See Chapter 10*
- Supported Butterfly (~10 minutes) *See Chapters 7 & 8*
- Supported Bridge (~10 minutes) *See Chapter 6*
- Savasana (~5 minutes) *See Chapter 11*
- Closing Pranayama: Balanced Breath (~5 minutes) *See Chapter 3*

BEFORE-BED RELAXATION SEQUENCE

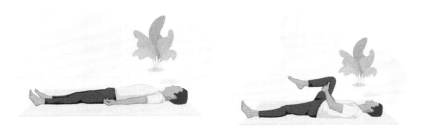

Knee-to-Chest Flow

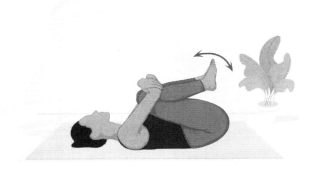

Low Back Massage Flow

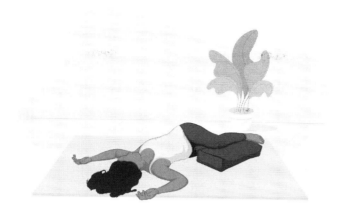

Supported Open Twist

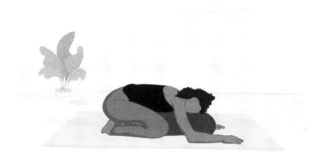

Sleeping Child's Pose

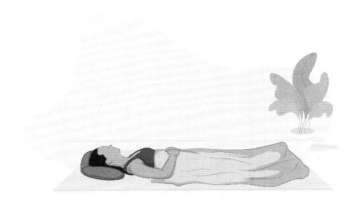

Corpse Pose

a. Purpose:

Use this pose before bed when you need a bit of help winding down. This sequence is designed to help those with insomnia or those who feel too wired to fall asleep. It also works well for people who simply want a pre-bed routine that is ready-made.

b. Duration:

45 minutes

c. Sequence:

- Pranayama: Three-Part Breath (~5 minutes) *See Chapter 3*
- Meditation: Progressive Muscle Relaxation (~5 minutes) *See Chapter 3*

- Warm-Up: (~5 minutes) *See Chapter 4*
- Knee-to-Chest Flow
- Low Back Massage Flow
- Supported Open Twist (~10 minutes total) *See Chapter 9*
- Sleeping Child's Pose (~10 minutes) *See Chapters 5, 7 & 9*
- Corpse Pose (~5 minutes) *See Chapter 7*
- Closing Pranayama: Balanced Breath (~5 minutes) *See Chapter 3*

SIMPLE SEQUENCE FOR HEADACHES AND MIGRAINES

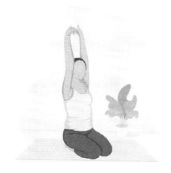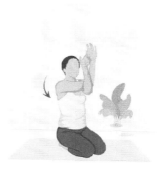

Eagle Arms Flow

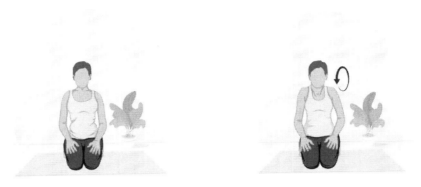

Shoulder Circles Flow

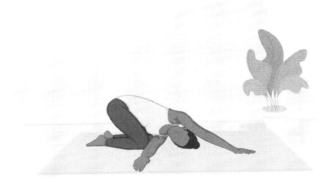

Thread the Needle

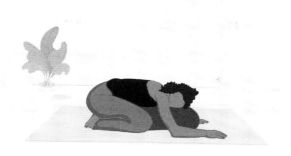

Child's Pose

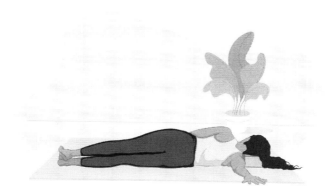

Front of the Shoulder Stretch

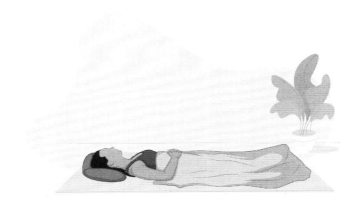

Corpse Pose

a. Purpose:

This sequence is designed to help you find relief from headaches and migraines as they arise. Every pose will help you find relief and restore balance to your body and mind. This sequence can be done with a cold compress for the eyes and forehead to provide additional relief from migraine symptoms.

b. Duration:

60 minutes

c. Sequence:

- Pranayama: Alternate Nostril Breath (~5 minutes)
  See Chapter 3

- Meditation: Progressive Muscle Relaxation (~5 minutes) *See Chapter 3*
- Warm-Up: (~5 minutes) *See Chapter 4*
- Eagle Arms Flow
- Shoulder Circles Flow
- Thread the Needle (~5 minutes each side; 10 minutes total) *See Chapter 5*
- Child's Pose (~15 minutes) *See Chapters 5, 7 & 9*
- Front of the Shoulder Stretch (~5 minutes each side; 10 minutes total) *See Chapter 6*
- Corpse Pose (~5 minutes) *See Chapter 7*
- Closing Pranayama: Alternate Nostril Breath (~5 minutes) *See Chapter 3*

HEALING FROM TRAUMA SEQUENCE

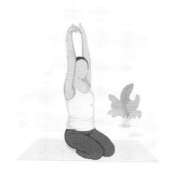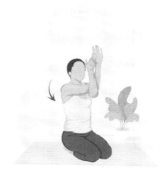

Eagle Arms Flow

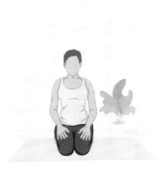
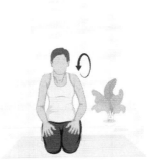

Shoulder Circles

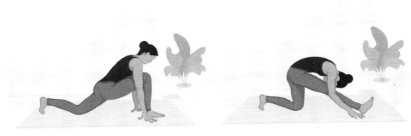

Low Lunge to Forward Fold Flow

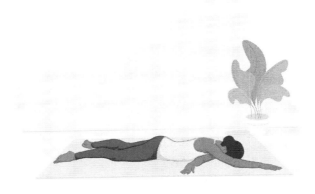

Thread the Needle

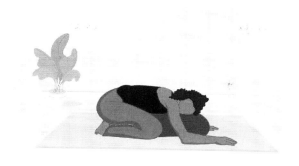

Child's Pose

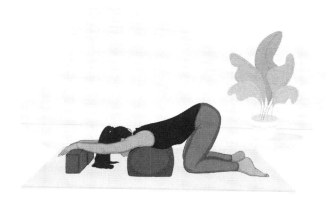

Melting Heart Pose

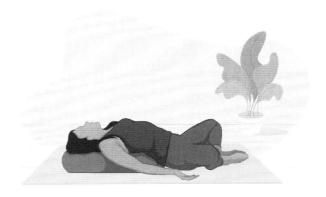

Supported Butterfly

a. Purpose:

This sequence is designed to help your body learn to self-regulate again in the wake of trauma. If you are someone with long-term PTSD or someone who recently went through a traumatic experience, this sequence is a great way to teach your nervous system that you are safe and ready to begin healing.

b. Duration:

    60 minutes

c. Sequence:

- Pranayama: Sitkari Breath (~5 minutes) *See Chapter 3*
- Meditation: Compassion for the Self (~5 minutes) *See Chapter 3*

- Warm-Up: (~10 minutes) *See Chapter 4*
- Eagle Arms Flow
- Shoulder Circles Flow
- Low Lunge to Forward Fold Flow
- Thread the Needle (~5 minutes each side; 10 minutes total) *See Chapter 5*
- Child's Pose (~10 minutes) *See Chapters 5, 7 & 9*
- Melting Heart Pose (~10 minutes) *See Chapters 5 & 6*
- Supported Butterfly (~5 minutes) *See Chapters 7, 8, 9 & 10*
- Closing Pranayama: Alternate Nostril Breath (~5 minutes) *See Chapter 3*

PRENATAL SEQUENCE FOR MAMAS-TO-BE

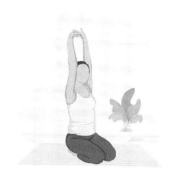 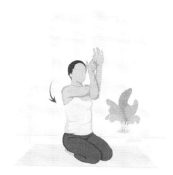

Eagle Arms Flow

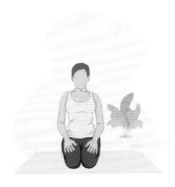
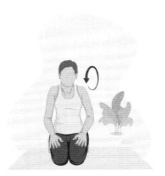

Shoulder Circles

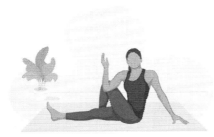
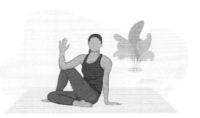

Flowing Seated Twists

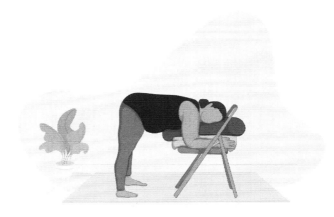

Wide-Legged Forward Fold with Chair

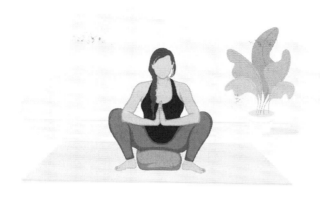

Supported Malasana

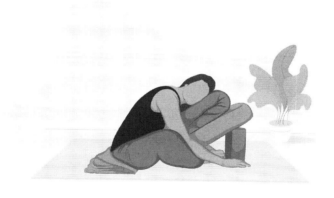

Supported Seated Butterfly

a. Purpose:

This sequence is designed for pregnant women to use throughout their pregnancy. Make sure that you speak with your healthcare provider before starting a new practice to ensure that you and your baby stay safe.

b. Duration:

45 minutes

c. Sequence:

- Pranayama: Balanced Breath (~5 minutes) *See Chapter 3*
- Meditation: Compassion (~5 minutes) *See Chapter 3*
- Warm-Up: (~5 minutes) *See Chapter 4*
- Eagle Arms Flow
- Shoulder Circles Flow
- Flowing Seated Twist
- Wide-Legged Forward Fold with Chair (~10 minutes) *See Chapter 9*
- Supported Malasana (~5 minutes) *See Chapter 9*
- Supported Seated Butterfly (~10 minutes) *See Chapter 9*
- Closing Pranayama: Apa Japa Breath (~5 minutes) *See Chapter 3*

CREATING YOUR OWN SEQUENCE

Creating your own sequence to follow is a fun way to begin playing around with your practice and making it your own. Consider the purpose of your flow and how you want to feel before selecting your pranayama, meditation, warm-up, and poses. Then, write down the elements of your sequence along with a rough estimate for timing.

When creating your own sequence, there is a simple formula to follow:

1. Pranayama
2. Meditation
3. Warm-Up
4. Poses
5. Closing Pranayama

Creating your own practice sequence can feel intimidating at first, but it doesn't have to be. If you are nervous about sticking to a plan or remembering your sequence, one strategy that I find helpful is writing my plan down on a piece of paper or a small whiteboard. This way, as I move from pose to pose, I can check in with my plan and make sure I'm not forgetting anything. With time, you will start to feel more confident and knowledgeable, eventually not requiring a written plan at all. Ideally, you will move toward a practice that flows intuitively from pose to pose as you take cues from your own physical needs and preferences.

Once you have developed a sequence that works well for you, take some time to repeat that sequence for a few days or even weeks. This will give you the space to get into a flow state where you no longer need to think about which poses come next. Once the sequence feels natural, sit with it for a while before adding something new.

Hopefully, this chapter has given you the tools to start building your own practice with knowledge and confidence. It's okay to stick to the practices I created for you, too, or to mix things up with some original and some preset sequences. Your main priority should be listening to your body and its needs. When you're not sure what to do, need some inspiration, or feel like you want to refresh your practice, this book will always be here for you as a resource.

LEAVE A QUICK REVIEW!

If you liked my book, I would greatly appreciate it if you could take 30 seconds to leave a review. Getting reviews helps this book reach more people like you, and it helps me know how I can best serve you. Thank you!

Scan the QR code to Leave A Quick Review

CONCLUSION

Now that you have completed this book, you should be well on your way to developing your own personal restorative yoga practice. One of the most valuable lessons I hope my readers take away is that restorative yoga is for everyone, regardless of your age, finances, gender, or physical abilities. You truly don't have to spend hundreds of dollars on props to create a healing, transformative practice in your life. This book, a few blankets and pillows, and a desire within you are truly all you need to begin implementing restorative yoga into your life. By taking the time to create a routine, you will give your mind, body, and spirit the gentle support it needs to flourish in all parts of your daily life. There is no replacement for rest and relaxation when it comes to your health.

My hope in writing this book is that you will keep it with you as a resource and a reference for your practice as you move through life. Yoga has been a thread throughout my life that has kept me feeling grounded, whole, and resilient. Passing on that feeling to my readers is an honor.

Yoga is a journey and sometimes it isn't a straightforward one. You might begin your practice right away, full speed ahead into a daily routine. Or, like me, you might practice a few times, then take a break when life gets complicated, only to rediscover restorative yoga again one day during an unexpectedly challenging time. Regardless of the path you take, when that time comes, I'll be here, ready to answer questions and help you find all of the amazing gifts that restorative yoga has to offer.

Now it's time for you to get started. Take a deep breath in and exhale, long and slow. Grab some cushions, blankets, towels, comfy clothes, and head to a quiet corner of your home for a quick restorative yoga session. Welcome to the incredible world of restorative yoga!

Namaste,

Mia

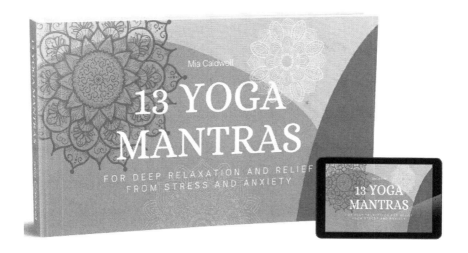

A FREE GIFT TO OUR READERS

Here is a list of my top 13 yoga mantras for relieving stress, free and ready to download right away! This will help you see noticeable results in your mindset, help you actually destress, and change the way you practice yoga forever. Visit this link to receive your gift:

www.miacaldwellbooks.com

RESOURCES

Ana, et al. "Elemental Rest: An Ayurvedic Approach to Restorative Yoga." Matthew Remski, 13 Sept. 2013, matthewremski.com/wordpress/elemental-rest-an-ayurvedic-approach-to-restorative-yoga/.

Art of Living Faculty. "The Practice: What Are the Eight Limbs of Yoga?" The Art of Living Retreat Center, 8 Jan. 2021, artoflivingretreatcenter.org/blog/practice-eight-limbs-yoga/

Ashtanga Yoga Girl, et al. "What Is Ashtanga Yoga? Everything You Need to Know!" Ashtanga Yoga Girl, 23 Mar. 2020, ashtangayogagirl.com/what-is-ashtanga-yoga/.

Bawden-Davis, Julie. "Restorative Yoga Poses for Back Pain." Parade, Parade: Entertainment, Recipes, Health, Life, Holidays, 27 Aug. 2020, parade.com/702782/juliebawden-davis/restorative-yoga-poses-for-back-pain/.

Beloved World Yoga. "Blog Detail." Yoga Studio in Jersey City, NJ, belovedworldyoga.com/restorative-yoga-poses-for-better-sleep/.

Bennett, Kate. "5 Best Yoga Poses to Help You Sleep Better and Relax at Bedtime." Calm Moment, 24 Mar. 2021, www.calmmoment.com/wellbeing/5-best-yoga-poses-to-help-you-sleep-better-and-relax-at-bedtime/.

Carr, Louise. "10 Reasons to Practice Restorative Yoga." DoYou, 2 Oct. 2014, www.doyou.com/10-reasons-to-practice-restorative-yoga/.

Clark, Sarah. "Can't Sleep? Try These 6 Restorative Poses Right in Bed." Yoga Journal, 27 Nov. 2017, www.yogajournal.com/poses/cant-sleep-6-restorative-yoga-poses-in-bed/.

Cook, Tracey. "Yoga and The Koshas - the Layers of Being." Ekhart Yoga, 13 Apr. 2020, www.ekhartyoga.com/articles/practice/yoga-and-the-koshas-the-layers-of-being.

Cronkleton, Emily. "10 Yoga Poses for Back Pain." Healthline, Healthline Media, 25 Aug. 2020, www.healthline.com/health/fitness-exercise/yoga-for-back-pain.

Cummins, Claudia. "Breathe to Relax in Restorative Yoga + Meditation." Yoga Journal, 28 Aug. 2007, www.yogajournal.com/practice/beginners/how-to/breathing-for-relaxation/.

Ekhart, Ester. "Restorative Yoga." Ekhart Yoga, 12 Aug. 2021, www.ekhartyoga.com/resources/styles/restorative-yoga.

Ferretti, Andrea. "Feel Happier: Poses for Depression & Anxiety." Yoga Journal, 27 Oct. 2007, www.yogajournal.com/lifestyle/feel-happier/.

The Good Body. "12 Benefits of Restorative Yoga: Relax and Start Healing." The Good Body, 12 Feb. 2021, www.thegood-body.com/benefits-of-restorative-yoga/.

Hanson, Rachel. "Yoga Visualization Practice." LoveToKnow, LoveToKnow Media, yoga.lovetoknow.com/Yoga_Visualization_Practice.

Harps, Carling. "8 Yin Yoga Poses to Relieve Low Back Pain." Alo Moves, 9 Aug. 2019, blog.alomoves.com/editors-picks/8-yin-yoga-poses-to-relieve-low-back-pain-3zzpp.

Harry. "Restorative Yoga Poses, Benefits and History." Yogi Weekly, 14 Nov. 2020, yogiweekly.com/restorative-yoga-poses-benefits-history/.

Heggs, Laura. "Rest and Digest: 8 Restorative Yoga Poses for Digestion." DoYou, 21 Oct. 2019, www.doyou.com/rest-and-digest-8-restorative-yoga-poses-for-digestion-91880/.

Hillary "20 Minute Restorative Yoga Flow for Neck Pain & Headaches." Jivayogalive, 12 Aug. 2019, jivayogalive.com/20-minute-restorative-yoga-flow-for-neck-shoulder-pain-and-headaches/

Hridaya Yoga. "Patanjali's Ashtanga Yoga the Eight Limbs." Hridaya Yoga, 23 Apr. 2021, https://hridaya-yoga.com/patanjalis-ashtanga-yoga-the-eight-limbs/

Johns Hopkins University. "9 Benefits of Yoga." Johns Hopkins Medicine, www.hopkinsmedicine.org/health/wellness-and-prevention/9-benefits-of-yoga.

Levine, Jessica. "5 Pranayama Techniques with the Power to Transform Your Practice-& Your Life." Yoga Journal, 17 June 2015, www.yogajournal.com/practice/importance-breath-yoga/.

Lindberg, Sara. "Restorative Yoga Poses: Benefits and Poses for Relaxation." Healthline, Healthline Media, 23 Sept. 2020, www.healthline.com/health/restorative-yoga-poses#benefits.

Lindberg, Sara. "What Are Chakras? Meaning, Location, and How to Unblock Them." Healthline, Healthline Media, 24 Aug. 2020, www.healthline.com/health/what-are-chakras#blocked-chakras.

Miller, Kelli. "What Is Ayurveda? Treatments, Massage, Diet, and More." WebMD, WebMD, www.webmd.com/balance/guide/ayurvedic-treatments.

Nair, Pritika. "9 Yoga Tips to Overcome Anxiety Disorder: Yoga Poses for Anxiety, Stress and Depression: Yoga Poses for Anxiety and Depression." Art of Living (Canada), www.artofliving.org/ca-en/yoga/health-and-wellness/yoga-for-anxiety-disorder.

Pizer, Ann. "How Restorative Yoga Can Improve Your Relaxation." Verywell Fit, www.verywellfit.com/what-is-restorative-yoga-3566876.

Ram. "Yin Yoga & Restorative Yoga: What Is The Difference?: Arhanta Yoga Blog." Arhanta Yoga Ashram, 16 July 2021, www.arhantayoga.org/blog/yin-yoga-versus-restorative-yoga-what-are-the-differences-and-similarities/

Raypole, Crystal. "Visualization Meditation: 5 Exercises to Try." Healthline, Healthline Media, 28 May 2020, www.healthline.com/health/visualization-meditation#goals-visualization.

Romine, Stepfanie. "Types of Yoga: A Guide to the Different Styles." Yoga Medicine, 13 Sept. 2019, yogamedicine.com/guide-types-yoga-styles/.

Rukat, Judy. "5 Types of Pranayama for Beginners." DoYou, 14 Feb. 2015, www.doyou.com/5-types-of-pranayama-for-beginners/.

Shah, Sejal. "Pranayama: The Top Beginner's Guide to Yoga Breathing Exercises." Art of Living (United States), www.artofliving.org/us-en/yoga/breathing-techniques/yoga-and-pranayama.

Simpson, Savitri. "Nine Deep Relaxations and Visualizations." The Expanding Light Retreat, www.expandinglight.org/free/yoga-teacher/advice/deep-relaxation.php.

Suni, Eric. "What Causes Insomnia?" Sleep Foundation, 6 Aug. 2020, www.sleepfoundation.org/insomnia/what-causes-insomnia.

West, Melissa. "Dosha Balancing Restorative Yoga: Ayurveda Yoga: Yoga with Melissa 450." Yoga Videos and Yoga Downloads., melissawest.com/450/.

Wikipedia. "Restorative Yoga." Wikipedia, Wikimedia Foundation, 19 July 2021, en.wikipedia.org/wiki/Restorative_Yoga.

Printed in Great Britain
by Amazon